Dear Barbara,
Dear Lynne

Dear Barbara,
Dear Lynne

The True Story of Two Women

in Search of Motherhood

Barbara Shulgold and Lynne Sipiora

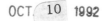

Addison-Wesley Publishing Company

Reading, Massachusetts Menlo Park, California New York Don Mills, Ontario Wokingham, England Amsterdam Bonn
Sydney Singapore Tokyo Madrid San Juan Paris Seoul Milan Mexico City Taipei

Library of Congress Cataloging-in-Publication Data

Shulgold, Barbara.
    Dear Barbara, dear Lynne : the true story of two women in search
of motherhood / Barbara Shulgold and Lynne Sipiora.
       p.   cm.
   ISBN 0-201-60841-3
   1. Sipiora, Lynne. 2. Childlessness—United States—Psychological
aspects—Case studies. 3. Infertility—United States—Psychological
aspects—Case studies. 4. Shulgold, Barbara. I. Sipiora, Lynne.
II. Title.
HQ536.S495 1992
306.874'3—dc20   92-8877
                                      CIP

Jacket design by Stephen Gleason
Text design by Barbara Cohen Aronica
Set in 11-point Berkeley Old Style by DEKR Corporation, Woburn, MA

1 2 3 4 5 6 7 8 9-MA-95949392
First printing, August 1992

For our sisters still waiting, and
for Lily, Tracey, and Destiny

Contents

Dear Barbara,
Dear Lynne

Searching

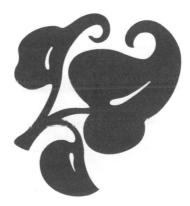

Lynne Sipiora was in her gynecologist's waiting room again. As she had done many times before, she flipped through the pile of magazines on the coffee table. But this time, something new caught her eye—a newsletter published by Resolve, the national organization for infertile people. She turned to the "Letters to the Editor" column and began to read . . .

RESOLVE NEWSLETTER,
FEBRUARY 1985

You are holding me . . .

It's 4:45 A.M. and my worst nightmare has awakened me to a real one—for the second time Perganol and we have failed. Once again I am not pregnant. I am trying to be brave through the cramps and, worse, the emotions. I need someone to comfort me, to stop the tears; but I am alone, my husband gone for the week.

So I turn to you. I reread the newsletter, as I have countless times, and magically, I am not alone. All of you who have shared this unique pain are holding me, and I am comforted.

How a simple eight-page newsletter has moved and strengthened me, consistently, month after month, is a never-ending source of amazement. To each of you who has ever written, thank you. You continue to be here when I need you.

Barbara Shulgold

MARCH 18, 1985

Dear Barbara,

I have not yet decided if I'm going to mail this letter or if I just need to write it for therapeutic reasons. Either way, the things you wrote in the *Resolve* newsletter touched me.

I had no idea there were people who felt as I do. The pain you described is something I consistently carry around and no one seems to understand. I have a wonderful husband, beautiful house, and exciting career but none of these things make up for the baby I may never have. Worse yet, I'm not even permitted to grieve.

If you have any interest in writing to me, please do so. I'm very interested in Pergonal and am slated to begin using it in another month. Also, I could use a "friend" who can really understand my sense of loss.

Wishing you success! (*Soon*)

Lynne Sipiora

MARCH 22, 1985

Dear Lynne,

I am pleased that you decided to mail your letter after all. I *am* interested in writing to you: I, too, could use a friend who understands my loss. I could use a sounding board—a place to express my deepest feelings. What safer person than a friend I don't know? I hope I can serve a similar purpose for you.

I wish I could be encouraging about Pergonal, but it didn't work for me. The letter you read in the February 1985 *Resolve* newsletter was written in October 1984, the month before our final try with Pergonal.

I have traveled miles and miles since then. When I finally gave up last November, I spent a rainy day home from work in bed, drinking wine and weeping and writing. I have spent hours and hours since then with Deborah, a nurturing and intuitive therapist. She helped me gather the courage to grieve and to say good-bye to the little girl I always believed I'd give birth to.

The grieving continues to be all-consuming. It is as if someone has died. Well, of course, there *has* been a death: the dream of a daughter who looks like me. And just like grieving death, grieving my loss has followed the classic stages: disbelief (denial), rage and then despair; I know the final stage is resolution, but I'm not there yet. I suffer bouts of hopelessness. I cry so often that I only remove my sunglasses at work. Nevertheless, I am getting better; I can feel it.

My greatest passion, my deepest secret since childhood has been my longing for motherhood. And a mother I will be! Rich (my husband) and I have initiated the adoption process. We will pursue open adoption. I don't know how long or hard *that* road will be; I only know we have chosen it. I for one will not stop traveling on it until we have reached our destination: a child.

In the meantime I must deal with a new source of grief and rage, and frankly, insane jealousy: Jennifer, an up-the-street neighbor (and fellow infertile), with whom I'm very good friends, is pregnant. She went to my infertility specialist who told her there was little chance she'd ever get pregnant. (I wonder if he had ever told *me* that if I would have gotten pregnant too!) In any case, even though I've gotten adept at avoiding seeing her growing tummy, I know it is nearby, and I feel affronted, mocked. C'mon fate, give me a break!

Please do write again soon. I look forward to hearing from you.

Barbara

APRIL 11, 1985

Barbara,

Thank you so much for responding to my letter and for sharing such personal feelings. It does indeed help to know that someone has been where I am. I think you're right about the stages of grief evoked by infertility following the stages of grief evoked by a death. I seem to be stuck in the stage of anger—anger at my total helplessness and anger at my body that just doesn't seem to work. Still, the anger is not as bad as the hurt.

Like you, since I was a little girl I have wanted a baby. As an adult, with a husband I love and a warm and secure marriage, the "want" has become a relentless need—I keep trying to understand the need—in hopes that that will be the key to controlling it. I know, I really do, that I am no less a person, no less a woman, without children. Nor do I think that babies *alone* make a fulfilling life, but even without any intellectual basis, I know I still "*need*." Everything I've always been tells me to continue to try—but when/if I must concede defeat, I don't know if I'll come out of it the same person. How do you give up a dream and carry on?

Barbara, I'm so sorry that you did not become pregnant. Frankly, your experience frightens me—because Pergonal is also my last resort. Still I'm glad you have initiated adoption because I can tell from your letter you possess all the sensitivity and caring needed to parent.

I know, all too well, how you feel about your neighbor's baby. Every time I hear about a friend or relative's pregnancy, I hurt. Sometimes I'm able to rationalize the envy away by telling myself it is not *their* baby or *their* experience that I want—therefore I am *not* jealous; it doesn't always work . . .

Thank you again for writing. It has truly helped me. There is so much more I would like to ask you and tell you—so I do hope that you'll write again.

By the way, when not obsessed with infertility I really am quite sane. I'm from Philadelphia but have been in the Chicago area ever since college. I'm thirty years old, the human resources manager of a large corporation, and a new owner of a house that needs lots of work. I mention all of that so you know there is more to me than my polycystic ovaries!

Thanks for caring.

Fondly,
Lynne

Dear Lynne,

Your letters have already become anticipated eagerly. They take some of my isolated feelings away, if only temporarily.

I've become absorbed with the notion of anger . . . since your first letter, actually. And I remember something I learned years ago, when I was in therapy: Depression is anger turned inward. It is *my* theory that women, feeling it's not "ladylike" to get angry, get depressed. It's a *lot* harder to deal with depression than anger. I was and am so frequently depressed over this issue. I rarely feel genuine rage.

All of which is my roundabout way of *encouraging* you to feel that anger (screwy, eh?). You will get through (past) it when you're ready. "Controlling it," which you say you want to do, might only put a lid on it . . . and then it would seep out, as depression.

You have a *right* to rage against life's blind unfairness; we both do. Will it "accomplish" anything concrete (like: a baby)? Of course not. But I feel it will help you to deal with all those strong feelings and free up energy to deal with what the immediate future holds.

Pergonal. Have you started? What schedule of follow-up tests will you have (ultrasounds? blood analysis?)? And *why* are you taking it? If it's because you don't ovulate when you take Clomid, you have an 80 percent chance of getting pregnant with the help of Pergonal. If you're taking Pergonal because of poor cervical mucus, you have a 50 percent chance of success. So, you see, the chances are good. But I still feel (for me) rational pessimism was the best way to deal with it. Otherwise the devastation can be crushing when a cycle fails.

I'd like to hear what you **are** doing to be good to yourself during your Pergonal cycles. Try to plan treats for yourself. We simplified our lives radically during my ovulation times: phone off the hook, dinners out (or delivered), quiet time. I can't urge you enough to try to eliminate as much stress from your life as you can. You can deal with stressful things later.

I enjoyed learning about the "other" you—career woman, etc.— in your final paragraph. And, I confess, it made me chuckle. There are still so many times when I find myself telling people (or myself) about the "other" me. Does it seem to you at times that a Person Trying to Get Pregnant is ALL there is to you? It's so consuming! There will come a day when you'll begin to get *bored* with the whole subject. That was a great day for me!

Here, I am getting ready for the scene of Barbara "oohing" and "aahing" over the baby due up the street in a couple of weeks. I can do it. Then I'll flop on the bed, cry, and then I'll go have a massage. And carry on.

I'm a teacher, so I'm off all summer. And Jennifer will be home with the baby. How am I going to deal with all this? I don't know.

A couple in our adoption group got a baby last month, and we recently met her. Lynne, a newborn baby is such a lovable, beautiful thing. *Any* baby. If you could have seen that baby, you too might have realized that having a baby come from your own body is secondary to *having a baby*. They are all precious. You . . . and I deserve that preciousness. And *we will have it*.

My best. Please write again.

Barbara Shulgold

MAY 5, 1985

Barbara,

Wonderful to receive your second letter—it arrived on the same day that I had a lengthy consult with my infertility specialist, so I suppose fate is *sometimes* on my side. I have not yet started Pergonal and probably will not for at least three more cycles. First I have to get rid of an infection I recently contracted, and then my doctor is insisting upon a *second* laparoscopy. She has an excellent reputation but is rather conservative in her approach. Though I'm anxious to get started, I'm also kind of relieved to be able to put it off for a while. Frankly, at this point I have no idea how I'll manage Pergonal. As you know, the Pergonal treatment requires going to the doctor for endless blood tests and ultrasounds during the first seven to twelve days of each menstrual cycle. My job requires me to travel, and my daily schedule is very unpredictable. I explained all of this to my doctor, and she said, "It's your choice." And so, once again I find myself angry! My career has been my salvation through all of this, and yet now I'm told rather plainly to choose between maintaining my career or risking it for a long shot on a baby. Actually there is no choice—I will opt for the latter and somehow or another work out the schedule—but *damn* it's just not fair!

Funny, but I knew you'd understand when I attempted to define the other me. I think I did it more for myself because I have to keep remembering that there *is* another me! Infertility *is* all consuming!

Re: adoption. Do you have any idea when you may get a baby? I am not opposed to the idea at all—but have been scared by a variety of stories on the unavailability of babies. Is this true? Are you going through an agency? How long have you been told you must wait? As usual, I have so many questions . . .

Know that I'll be thinking of you as your neighbor's baby arrives on the scene. I face a similar situation. My husband has a nine-year-old daughter from a previous marriage. She is a sweet kid and we get along well—but she is *not* mine. Ann is with us every other weekend, and sometimes just looking at her is difficult. I find myself consumed with jealousy that my husband was able to have a child with another woman, but not with me! From time to time she asks very normal questions about when she was born, and when Ken tells the story of the trip to the hospital, etc., I really cannot bear it! I had not intended to get into yet *another* of my problems, but somehow I think you'll understand.

You're right—the statistics on Pergonal are encouraging, but like you, I am cautious. Ovulation *and* cervical mucus are a problem for me—the ultimate double whammy! While I await Pergonal, I continue to take 100 milligrams of Clomid a day for five days per month, and I continue to hope. Despite many, many disappointments, I continue to feel symptoms of pregnancy—every month—right up to the day my period arrives. Crazy, I know.

I've tried to take your advice about being good to myself and it does help. I also talk to no one (except Ken) about my problem—I think that helps me keep it in perspective. Also, I could not stand the monthly requests for progress reports. I did speak to my mother once, who only said, "Oh well you're a career woman, not the maternal type anyway." Needless to say, we've not discussed it again. I think that's why writing to you has become very important—not only do I feel free to say exactly what I feel but, wonder upon wonder, you know what I'm talking about. Yes, Barbara, there just are not many people who can intelligently talk cervical mucus and the luteal phase—pity to be so uninformed! The last line of your recent letter confirmed what I've always believed—I do *deserve* a baby. I know you do too. I will anxiously await all the details of your soon-to-arrive "preciousness," because I feel confident that when that baby is in your arms you'll be able to put all of this aside. I hope I, too, have such a happy ending. I also hope I end up half as well adjusted as you are!

Keep in touch. My thoughts are with you.

Lynne

P.S. I *hate* Mother's Day!

MAY 12, 1985
Just another Sunday
(Really. That's all it is.)

Dear Lynne,

Your "P.S. I hate Mother's Day!" rang true for me. Up to this year I'd thought of it as free publicity for the Hallmark Corporation and shrugged it off. But, because I want a baby so much right now, today is harder. So I decided to do something about it.

First, I tried to get the women in my adoption group to join me for brunch. Although only one could make it, we did have a fine time commiserating. (This resilient woman has had four miscarriages and two stillbirths and is an obstetrics nurse!!) You were toasted in tea, and certainly thought of.

Then when my traditional Sunday radio show (bluegrass) asked for Mother's Day requests, I got inspired. I called and asked them to play something cheery for all infertile women, for whom this day was hard. (Hold on now.) The song they chose: "It's Too Late." I slammed out of the house so I wouldn't hear it. So many people are ignorant, ignorant, *ignorant* about what infertility means; no wonder we are guarded with our stories and our sadness. Sometimes, all of this makes me so tired and I despair.

I felt you were thinking of me when I learned Friday that the couple up the street had a healthy girl. Let me tell you, if bad wishes could cause birth defects, that should've been one messed-up kid. You know I don't even feel guilty writing that; there's a lot of anger still left in me, I think.

You'd have been proud of me as I trudged my way up the street to deliver the soft stuffed polar bear I'd bought. (I bought *two*—one for my future baby, too!) I smiled at them and said all the appropriate things (haven't seen the baby yet—that'll be a toughy). Then walked back down the street and asked Rich for a long hug while I shook and cried.

We women certainly are trained to be gracious ("ladylike"). Is that why I could pull off such a totally phony scene? And why you don't know what to do with the anger? ("Ladies" don't get angry; it's not nice.)

I have searched the house looking for a recent *Ms.* magazine that focused on stepfamilies because I think it included an article on being a stepparent and infertile. Can't find it, but if I do, I'll send it right out. You would be comforted, I think, to hear another woman expressing her jealousy of her husband's being able to produce a child, of her feelings of isolation . . . partly from him because he didn't understand; he'd *already* reproduced himself.

To have your infertility thrown in your face when your stepdaughter visits every two weeks sounds rough. Can you make anything positive out of it? (You certainly are more in touch with the day-to-day reality of parenting, I'll bet!) I give you my support.

It sounds like you and I have exactly the same medical problems. Was your mucus problem caused by cervicitis, too? When will the laparoscopy be, and why does your doctor feel you need another? Endometriosis?

Now then, this is *important:* I had no idea you knew so little about independent (or "private") adoption. Herewith a brief explanation which will make the "last resort" not such a hopeless one.

I'll bet the reason you seem to know little about private adoption is that it's illegal in your state. *But that doesn't mean you can't do it.*

We have a local adoption lawyer who has explained all the ins and outs to us. Basically, you send out 1,000 to 2,000 resume-like letters to ob/gyns, family practice doctors, lawyers, etc., as well as people in your personal network. And then you wait. The *average* waiting time is seven to twelve months! And it works: I know three couples who've gotten babies that way in the last six months (longest wait = twelve months).

It's also expensive ($4,000 to $6,000). I inherited about that much from my aunt's death last year, so it's become our adoption fund.

It's legal.

And, it's risky. The birthmother can change her mind before the birth or up to six months after (depending on state laws), although this happens in only 5 to 10 percent of the cases.

You, with the help of your lawyer, do the negotiating and that's hard. But for most couples, there's no other option.

I'll be happy to write you more about private adoption if you have other questions.

But I do have a slightly bizarre suggestion: Why don't you and your husband register at adoption agencies now? The wait may be four years, but by then you may be open to adopting a second child, regardless of how you got the first one. The disadvantage with agencies is that with most of them you have no direct contact with the birthmother. (You usually do contact the birthmother when you adopt privately.) The advantage is that going through an agency is less risky, because there are tighter legal controls, making it harder for the birthmother to change her mind.

I really wish I could offer encouragement about coordinating work and Pergonal. But until this society puts life before profit, well . . . you get my drift. I wasted six precious months last year waiting to do Pergonal in the summer when I don't teach so that all the required doctor's visits wouldn't be so hard to schedule. Ha! It slipped into six cycles anyhow, and doing it in September, at the start of the year, was murder.

I hope your boss is someone you can level with. I hope there is flexibility there (could you work overtime on the days you don't go to the doctor?). Just one thing I really want to say: You obviously are clear about your priorities. *Don't let job pressures guilt-trip you off the track.*

More to come. More to say. But all this has tired me. I'm still a bit frazzled from dealing with the folks up the street.

I look forward to your next letter.

Barbara

MAY 21, 1985

Barbara,

Received your recent letter with picture and was amazed to see that you look exactly as I'd imagined.

Mother's Day was not quite as bad as I'd anticipated, but last weekend was horrible. We invited several couples with their children to our home for a picnic. Annie, Ken's daughter, was also with us for the weekend. The entire afternoon was spent on discussions of parenting, home vs. work, pregnancy, delivery—well you get the picture. Finally, at six o'clock, the group broke up. Ken drove his daughter home to her mother, and I went to my bedroom and fell apart. I cried for at least an hour, then went downstairs, brought a bottle of wine to my bed, and cried some more. At that moment I decided I really couldn't stand any of those people, and I was not even too crazy about Ken. *Everyone* it seems has a baby but me! I don't know if I can, or even should, attempt to explain how awful it was—but in retrospect, I seem to have gone over the edge. When Ken returned, he said all of the usual "comforting things," and suddenly even he sounded patronizing and condescending, and I decided there is no one who understands—except maybe you. As usual, I recovered—got to my office early and continued to pull off my competent, in-control-career-lady routine. How is it that we are so resilient?

Treatment continues—during May my lab work and ultrasounds will be repeated. It now appears Pergonal may start in July. I will definitely have to talk to my boss. He's a pretty good guy, but the subject is one I'm not anxious to share with him. Should he be accommodating so I can get pregnant and resign? It's all very complicated. Still, I'm hopeful I can curtail travel and just do it. How long do people usually keep taking Pergonal? Did your husband give you the injections? Did you have any side effects? I'm frightened but very hopeful, always hopeful . . . I don't know why I have a mucus and ovulation problem—nor does my doctor. She seems to feel that my hormone level is the main source of the problems, but she's not pinpointed anything to date.

Sorry, so sorry about the neighbor's baby. Have you had to see her yet? If I were you, I would really try to keep my distance from the entire scene throughout the summer. The information on adoption was fascinating—you are right; I knew nothing. I also agree with your suggestion about going to an agency *now*, but Ken is not ready yet— and may never be—I don't know.

As usual, much to say. My letters to you have become a form of therapy, I think, and your responses are very important. How wonderful to have a summer off—what are your plans? Are you taking your own advice of being good to yourself? I hope so.

Lynne

JUNE 5, 1985

Dear Lynne,

I have just a quiet hour to write to you before I return to the high-pressure madness of the last two weeks of school. A few moments ago I had just settled into a chair on the porch, when there, a few yards up the hill, was Jennifer with her baby girl. I am pretending (*hard*) that you are here listening to me as, slowly, the reality of finally seeing a real baby sinks in. That was the moment I've been dreading for nine months. As usual, not as bad as I feared; it is, after all, just a baby— i.e., not *my* baby. I wanted to caress the softness of her cheeks and feel her warmth, but I looked away, chatted amiably (I'm so *great* at that b.s.), and came in. Damn, Lynne, here come the tears.

Time out.

The song on the bluegrass record I'm playing is "No One Knows" (the inward grief of my poor troubled mind). Not true: We know each other's, and right now I am so grateful for that knowledge.

On this end, much continued resolute courage as I wait and wait and wait—courage needed because the woman whom I've gone through all this with, from my Resolve infertility support group, just brought home an adopted baby girl. It took ten months incidentally, a bit longer than normal around here for private adoption. So you (and I) should take heart from that. And in two weeks the surrogate baby of a friend in Los Angeles is due. I am very happy for her. But oh, jealousy and renewed panic as I edge closer to forty-two. Be grateful you aren't my age; every month makes me feel so old, useless, hopeless, *wasted* (and wondering: Can I raise two kids in my mid-forties? We hope to adopt two eventually).

I appreciate your advice about keeping my distance from the baby up the street. I intend to follow it. But I'm no longer going to avoid the porch, as I have the past year. I love to sit over the yard in the sun in the summer and read or write or whatever. I consider that being good to myself. And I think I can deal with the baby now. The worst was today when I *had* to notice her. Sometimes it helps to say, "It's just ——————," whether it's a feeling ("It's just sadness") or a baby or a pang of rage . . . well, you know. Try it; it might work for you, too.

My adoption group was here for a potluck Sunday. I told everyone (fourteen of us) about you. And we all agreed we have it easier because we have each other. (Idea: Could you try to contact Resolve and start a support group? Aren't you near a big city?) One couple in my group is pregnant—and we all agreed it was great not to feel jealous. One has an adopted baby, Megan (it took eight months and 1,500 letters). One is considering international adoption. Three couples, including us, are trying for private adoption. We are determined to keep meeting until there are six screaming brats around us! (One couple will be returning to their native Switzerland next year and will then probably pursue international adoption, the *only* realistic option in Europe, incidentally.)

I almost called you when the Frustace septuplets hit the news. I could just imagine how freaked out it must have made you. It made

me *furious!* It's irresponsible medicine for a specialist to monitor Pergonal dosage so carelessly that seven eggs would be fertilized. My
gynecologist (on the board of directors of Resolve, by the way) told
me over a year ago that doctors and clinics that get women in such a
position are flaky. I agree. Part of the Pergonal procedure includes
frequent ultrasounds, used to check on the growth of egg follicle(s).
One cycle, I had three ripe follicles, and against everyone's advice, I
refused to be "ovulated." I didn't want to take the chance of having
triplets if all three "took." When the doctor said that I could always
abort, I came close to hitting him. I believe in a woman's right to
choose, but do you think I'd have had an abortion after three years of
trying to get pregnant? No way! I'll always wonder what would have
happened if I'd chosen to continue that cycle.

Mrs. Frustace was clearly given way too high a dosage of Pergonal.
There is really no excuse for that. If you've continued to follow the
story in the papers, you may have read an article that said essentially
that the clinic she went to was doing careless work. If you trust your
doctor's expertise, you have nothing to fear. Boy, though, it still
infuriates me just writing about it. I hate to think how it must have
affected you.

You asked about Pergonal's side effects: not a lot, compared to
Clomid (are you taking that now?). Around ovulation time, Pergonal
creates tons of discharge. No big deal—in fact, I kind of liked it
because it made me feel I was establishing the right environment for
sperm.

Also, your ovaries get highly stimulated, so my doctor said no
exercise during the second half of the cycle—a real drag, as I had to
drop my aerobics class (one of my sources of sanity) for six months.
You may feel the enlarged ovaries. I often felt swollen inside and
sensitive. A jarring action hurt, so I was just careful not to bound
downstairs—things like that. Mostly, the side effects were bearable.
Much harder was the way it all just absorbed our lives—*totally.*

I understand too well the scene during and after all the "parents"
(and Ken) left. I won't even tell you how many times *I've* crawled into
bed with brandy (my drug of choice) and wept. I don't know how
you feel, but it seemed so familiar to me. You should have seen me

the day I heard Jennifer (my up-the-street neighbor) was pregnant!! But, Lynne, I survived it . . . and you will too.

They don't understand. Ken (and Rich) don't either. It doesn't mean they don't care, though. Ken, like Rich, is clearly doing the best he knows how. Take whatever he has to offer, but don't expect him to meet your needs. Can't be done. Spread it out—to him, to me, to a therapist, to anyone who can try to help. No one person can be all to you that you need right now. But every little bit will help.

And, continuing my motto of being good to yourself: Why do you *have* to be part of such a scene? During my worst of times, Rich went off to many social events without me and made excuses. Too many moms or babies for me to handle. No one said you have to be stoic/masochistic/"brave." Screw it. This *won't* go on forever, even though it sure can feel like it. Take care of yourself *now*. If they call you antisocial, you have two choices: (1) tell them the truth or (2) let them.

And answers to other Pergonal questions: Doctors usually recommend trying Pergonal for three cycles, but sometimes as many as six, as in my case, because some eggs have to be "aborted" (hmph!) midcycle for a variety of reasons, usually concerning your health. I wish it were more cut and dried, for the sake of your sanity *and* your work, but it's not. Yes, my husband gave me the injections. It's very easy, except for the first time. I usually watched TV while he did it, because if you're nervous your muscles tighten up and it hurts more. The good news is it will draw Ken more into the process, and you will feel less alone.

Well, Lynne, I'm thinking of you. I genuinely like our correspondence and look forward to hearing from you. Let's continue to "use" each other as a sounding board. We can say *anything* in our letters and that *is* therapeutic!

Best wishes,
Barbara

P.S. Why don't *you* send a photo so *I* can see if you look as *I* imagine?

JUNE 14, 1985

Barbara,

I'm writing today from my doctor's waiting room—which somehow seems very appropriate. There are five other women seated here, but we don't look at each other and never speak. Whenever I am in this situation, I have this fantasy of getting up from my seat, standing on the coffee table, where the dated *House Beautifuls* are kept, and screaming "*I'm mad as hell and I'm not going to take it anymore!*" Then all the other women also jump to their feet and join me in the chant. Together we push our way past the bitchy receptionist and break down the door of the doctor's office. Then we physically remove her from her desk and tie her to the examining table (stirrups optional). We refuse to release her until she "cures" each of us—at which point, of course, she does. As you see, my rage has begun to take on some violent overtones—but they are strictly limited to fantasy, because in reality I am oh-so-very polite—even to the bitchy receptionist!

My appointment is now over, and once again Pergonal has been postponed. This time my doctor has requested that Ken have a hamster penetration test to see if his sperm can penetrate an egg and that I undergo another series of ultrasounds to check follicle production. I will, of course, do as I'm told, but I am so anxious to get on with it. Yes, I am currently on Clomid (150 milligrams per day now) and a steroid called Cecadron. I've experienced no side effects with any of these drugs and, physically, feel fine. Your description of Pergonal treatment was reassuring, and I *am* ready—maybe in July . . .

Last Saturday evening I had an interesting experience. Ken and I went to dinner with a couple we know, but not well. They are in their early thirties, married four years, with no children. Well, somehow their childless status came up, and the woman said (very matter-of-factly), "We have no children because I am infertile—I discovered a few years ago that I have an ovulation problem." I was amazed at her candor and thrilled to perhaps have stumbled upon a kindred spirit. "Are you being treated for it?" I asked, and she said, "No, I assume it's just meant to be." Then I said (despite the fact that Ken was kicking me under the table), "How does that make you feel?" And she said,

"Well, I was surprised and disappointed, but there are worse things that could happen." That was the end of the discussion, but I kept thinking how very amazing her reaction was. Here I am losing my mind, crying three or four times daily and going to bed with wine bottles, and she says, "La-de-da—what will be, will be." I think if you and I had not been writing, I would have surely determined at that point that I am *stark, raving, mad.* Thank you (again and again) for making me feel less alone.

Glad your experience with the baby up the street was not as bad as anticipated. My brother's baby was born two weeks ago—right on schedule—and I practiced your technique of "It's only jealousy" and it *did* help.

How exciting that your friend got a baby and that it *can't* be too much longer until you do. Have you had responses from your letters? How many have you sent out? I really feel as though you'll be successful, and I am hoping for you every day. Do keep me posted.

Your advice re: Ken not meeting *all* of my needs was timely. I find myself getting so frustrated with him sometimes because "he doesn't know how I feel" . . . I must remember that he is a loving and sensitive man, and he is doing the best he knows how. Do you feel infertility has strengthened your relationship? From your letters it appears that it has. Perhaps one day when I can be more objective, I will really be able to understand the effect it has had on us. One final thought that perhaps you can lend some understanding to—I've decided that I am embarrassed about being infertile and that is why I can't discuss it. I don't think I'd be embarrassed about high blood pressure or diabetes or anything else out of my control, but this is how I feel. I guess I'm afraid that if anyone knew they'd pity me, and I can't bear the thought of that. Have you felt this way? Must close— flying out tonight to Oklahoma City for a business meeting. Time to put on my well-balanced, career woman routine and perform accordingly. I will try to find a photo before I send this.

Take good care,
Lynne

JULY 7, 1985

Lynne,

Oh no! June 14 is the date of your last letter. I'm sorry to have taken so long, but it was also the last day of school, and I invariably collapse for a couple of weeks after that. It felt wonderful to just vegetate and not be "Ms. Shulgold" any more.

Your doctor office fantasy had me in stitches. Yes, I know, it's not really funny . . . but what else can we do? I identified with your rage. I can't even drive by my doctor's building without breaking out in an icy rage. By the way, I think all infertility specialists must intentionally hire bitchy receptionists. Mine was Ms. Ice Heart of '85. I guess they want to diffuse our rage by diverting our attention to the rudeness of their receptionists.

None-of-my-business-but department: The hardest part of infertility for me/us was lack of control. I can sense your similar frustration. So, what would it feel like to set some time limits (on your doctor and maybe even on you): I will try Pergonal if ———— doesn't happen by ———— (date). If the Clomid doesn't get me pregnant by ————, then . . . It's your body, dammit. (I get angry just imagining what you're feeling.) You are not a bitch by taking some control away from your doctor; you are just taking care of yourself. I bet setting limits will reduce some of your anger, too. You're probably healthily assertive on the job; aren't your life and your body more important? Sermon for the day completed.

The woman whose attitude was "What will be, will be" struck me as a bit odd. Either she really didn't want children, or she can't cope with the pain. I don't buy her response. I wonder what would have happened if the two men (Ken and her husband) hadn't been there. I'll bet you'd have heard something else!

So now I'm looking at your paragraph about the baby up the street and feeling that what I wrote about my feelings is only sometimes true—I continue to take your advice about keeping my distance, but what can I tell you? Rich and I have been working in the yard all day—I *love* putting my hands in soil and making things grow. Every time I'd glance up and see those baby things on the clothesline almost *hanging over* me . . . the irony of my trying to make something grow while a woman who won't pinch a tomato off a vine (really!) hangs up baby things . . . well, I, too, could scream with you I CAN'T STAND IT; I WON'T TAKE ANY MORE!!

But there are days when I hear the kid scream and scream and *scream,* and I'm not so sure I'm discontented after all. There's nothing like a good dose of reality.

You asked about my adoption hopes. I guess we've been corresponding for a shorter time than I realized (short but intense, yes?), and I never told you about the Texas baby. We sent out over 600 letters January 27 and got our "magic" phone call February 6 about a teacher (!) seven months pregnant who wanted to give up the baby. Ah, Lynne, I can barely write this (I thought you knew). Insane, youthful chaos ensued. We went on a baby-things buying spree, chose names, read tons of books on child care, lost our ability to sleep, and told *everyone* (yes, up the street, too). Friends began planning a shower.

Two weeks before her due date she decided to keep her baby. (It was her baby all along—not meant to be mine.) I crumbled. I was hysterical for over a week—cried in my *class,* for Pete's sake, and spent much time in bed with brandy (sound familiar?). Rich was totally helpless. I don't believe I could have made it without my super therapist. Lynne, it was then I learned that this *can* happen in private adoption—a birthmother can change her mind about giving up her baby. (Almost everyone has it happen at least once.) Once again, fate demands strength we never knew we'd need.

It toughened me. So when the second call came, I was in a very different place. That's an equally long and somewhat painful story. Basically, a woman claiming to be Jewish said she wanted to give us her child because I'm also Jewish. She was married with two kids already—could we help move the family from Texas to California? Set them up in an apartment? (Get the picture?) We were 90 percent certain it was a scam and turned them down cold. An even more appalling fact than that birthmothers change their minds is the fact that there are con artists out there. Bastards—taking advantage of our desperation! We were glad that it wasn't our first phone call.

It was the good, healthy feeling I got after saying no to that woman that made me realize that taking as much control as possible over this essentially uncontrollable situation (infertility and/or adoption) was what would help me make it through. Thus my sermon of pages one and two.

We've sent out 2,000 letters to doctors and are now beginning to ask everyone in our personal and work networks to give our letters and photos to any counselors, teachers, or doctors they might know. (Fifty percent of babies are found this way.)

My original Resolve infertility group has dwindled down to two couples still hoping for babies.

So last week we got a phone call from Colorado. There's a seventeen-year-old there deciding whether to give up her baby, due in September, to Catholic Social Services or us. Why am I so very pessimistic/unexcited? I'm protecting myself. I don't dare get excited; the thought of that disappointment again is too painful. I'll let you know.

You asked about the effect of infertility on our marriage. Man, you wouldn't believe what *that* started! I asked Rich what *he* thought and out came anger, hurt, pain. We started to talk about it and began fighting like we hadn't done in years. Of course, *you're* not responsible, but I thought you'd be interested.

Rich held it all in and tried his mightiest to support me during those long worst-of-times. Now that I am feeling far less grief-stricken, his guard is down. So we're going through a lot now: We agreed that he needed to relearn expressing his anger; thus, there are lots of arguments.

Will we make it? Yes. Is our relationship stronger? I think so. I also wonder if we'll *ever* get over all of it, if we'll ever be the same. I doubt it. I feel in Rich's debt, and he feels short-changed. It's going to take a while. There is no question infertility profoundly affects marriages. (I've participated in two studies through the University of California Medical Center and Resolve that came to that conclusion.) No man can ever understand a woman's grief over an inability to conceive, and no woman can understand what that loss feels like to a man.

You asked about feeling embarrassed about infertility. I am wiped out, as usual. These letters require a lot and I need to stop now. Ask me again in your next letter, OK?

I don't know the answers. I'm not sure there are any—certainly not easy ones. I *do* know that you strike me as honest, stronger than you realize (all of this *is* strengthening you), and smart. You'll make it through—that sounds simplistic, but you will because the alternative is unthinkable.

Mmm. I'm getting incoherent. More very soon. I'm going to the Vancouver Folk Festival July 11–July 17 and will see my dear friend Eva in Vancouver and have fun and forget for a while. I'll try to send you a card.

My thoughts are with you.

Barbara

P.S. You forgot your photo.

JULY 31, 1985

Barbara,

Just returned from a week-long family reunion in Ocean City, New Jersey. This is an annual event where all of the siblings return to the ancestral manse, hug and kiss one another to death, and then, very soon after, start to fight. Invariably someone leaves in a snit, only to return the following year and repeat the entire cycle—ah, *tradition!*

Re: your last letter. I had no idea about all of the adoption traumas you've been through to date. Your consistent strength never ceases to amaze me. Since my last letter, I have had my own share of trauma. In June I took my usual Clomid, then had ultrasounds and was inseminated and, wonder upon wonder, did *not* get my period when expected. It was fifteen days late when I finally called the doctor, and despite my best defenses, I was wildly optimistic. My breasts were tender, I was throwing up every morning, and I swear I even looked at wallpaper for a nursery. A pregnancy test was scheduled for yesterday morning at 9:00 A.M.—well, of course, you know how this ends. I awoke at 6:00 A.M. with terrible cramps and my period, and I really felt I was going to just die of disappointment. I cried through the entire day, drank most of a bottle of wine that night, and awoke today—better. How is it that we are so resilient—over and over again?

More and more, adoption appears the only alternative. I have decided I will not continue treatment past Christmas 1985—I just can't deal with it longer than that.

Sorry my question on infertility and marriage dragged up some unresolved issues. I mentioned it because I've already been there. Like Ken, I too was married before. My ex-husband and I were treated together for infertility for awhile and divorced when we finally gave up on that and each other. I am often afraid that treatment will come between Ken and me, but I think the difference this time is that I will *not* sacrifice a husband for a baby.

I want to ask you about your adoption progress, but I'm not sure that I should. I often resent friends who ask me for an update; still other times I'm hurt when they do not. So anyway, tell me how you feel about this.

Vancouver sounds wonderful—a great respite from the usual. What else are you doing this summer—for you? Well, I must wrap this up for now. I think of you so often!

Lynne

P.S. Finally managed to dig up a photo from last Christmas. I'd like to tell you that we're much better looking in real life, but as they say, "The camera never lies . . ."

AUGUST 12, 1985

Dear Lynne,

I am still basking in the afterglow of a wonderfully relaxing time in Vancouver. I spent three days lolling on the grass, listening to all kinds of folk music. I promised myself this would be a *real* vacation, that I would leave my infertility behind in another country. And as much as it is possible to play such a psychological trick on myself, I succeeded. It's amazing how ready-for-anything I feel right now. The healing effects of a vacation cannot be underrated. In fact, infertility specialists should *prescribe* them!

You wondered if it's all right to ask about the adoption process. Remember, we promised each other that this would be a no-holds-barred correspondence. Let's not trip ourselves up with "good manners," which might only succeed in keeping us from saying what we need to say and asking what we need to ask. . . . Anyhow, what else would I write about—the weather? politics?

Returning home to learn that the Colorado teenager did not choose us hardly threw me. Maybe Vancouver's restorative powers are still strong, and I can let the loss go. Or maybe I am getting used to failure. Or maybe on some level I am coming to accept that there are dues (failures—"leads that fall through," they are called) to be paid. In any case, I feel emotionally ready to endure whatever lies ahead . . . until I am a mother.

In the midst of this frustrating time, it is easy to lose sight of what we've got going for ourselves. We *are* strong. We have survived plenty already, not even counting infertility. We are also damn funny; don't ever discount the curative value of humor. And, we have the invaluable ability to reach out to others for renewal!

But being strong, open, and funny won't find you your baby. Keep covering your bases; start researching adoption now. Maybe it will prove unnecessary, but "it couldn't hoit," as my mother would say.

Enough. Time to get out in the sunshine before it's back-to-school time again.

Love,
Barbara

AUGUST 26, 1985

Barbara,

I've taken your advice and started researching adoption. As usual, there is good and bad news. On the down side, every Illinois agency has a waiting list of at least *five* years. Further, 50 percent of them would not even consider us eligible to "wait" because Ken has a "natural" child! Can you believe it? The good news is that private adoption was legalized here in 1983. I've been referred to an attorney who will provide more information, and I plan to call him soon.

"Covering emotional bases" . . . you're right, it makes sense. August was a tense month in regard to my ongoing treatment. Despite a few new wonder drugs, I had yet another poor postcoital test. So, even though it was good for me and good for Ken, it wasn't good enough for anything else! It has been decided that insemination will now become part of the monthly routine—I had my first one last Saturday. It seems to me that there has got to be a flaw in my treatment—ultrasound confirms follicle development with Clomid; insemination assures that the sperm get where they are supposed to, when they are supposed to. So what is missing? I guess as we continue, we will find out. Isn't it amazing that anyone ever *accidentally* gets pregnant?

Did I tell you I told my parents about my infertility? My main reason for doing so was to stop the baby-related inquiries, and that I have done. But now I find I am on the receiving end of a million infertility stories. It seems just about everyone my mother has ever known was told they'd never get pregnant, tried for years and years, and then ta-da—to the amazement of their doctors and friends—had a baby. The best story to date is of a woman who was told she'd never conceive and was, naturally, devastated. Still, she carried on. After fifteen years of marriage, at age forty-five, she was in a terrible auto accident. They pulled her, barely alive, from the rubble, and the very next month she got pregnant. "So what's the point, Mother?" I stupidly asked. "Well," she replied, "obviously the accident jarred her body into functioning." Interesting clinical assessment, don't you think? Care to go for a spin and ram ourselves into a tree?

Your last letter's optimism was good for me—as is every letter you've written. You are a living, breathing example of hope—hope that no matter what happens, I will be okay. Someday maybe I will provide the same hope for someone else. It's a mitzvah (and here you thought I was a Waspy midwesterner; actually, I guess I am, but I was madly in love with a very observant Jew once, and our romance left me with a lot of interesting, though basically useless, information). Thanks also for reconfirming my strength. I *am* strong, though I tend to forget from time to time.

Perhaps being a teacher, you feel as I do—that the year starts in September. The end-of-summer change of season always feels more like a beginning to me than January. So I hope our years go well, and I really believe that they will.

Remember, I'm thinking of you and hoping for you!

Lynne

SEPTEMBER 10, 1985

Dear Lynne,

Yes, September always feels like the start of the year to me, both as a Jew and as a teacher. I heard an inspiring sermon on "Beginnings" in temple on Rosh Hashanah and was enthusiastically ready to begin a new year and a new class at school . . . but then those thirty shining faces stared back at me from their seats on the first day of school— my seventeenth year, for Pete's sake—and I remembered: I don't want to be doing this anymore. I don't want to be *in loco parentis* for other people's children (some of whom are other people's mistakes, brought into the world and raised by accident). I want to be the parent of *my* children and make *my* mistakes.

Thanks for relating your mother's story of the woman who got pregnant the month after her dreadful car accident. I will indeed gladly join you for that spin into a tree . . . provided *your* car carries good insurance.

Isn't it amazing the silly things people (usually, well-meaning female friends and relatives) will say to encourage you? My favorite is, "Go ahead and adopt. I know this woman who did and got pregnant the very next month!" Facts are that only 7 percent of women who adopt then go on to get pregnant and carry babies to term. But hey, when throwing that back in the face of a woman I know, I heard, "Seven percent? That's not bad odds." Uh huh.

Actually, I am close to being finished with all that. Day by day I am clearer and clearer that I have abundant love to give a child. I am anxious for that child to arrive; it is less and less important *how* he or she gets here. All that grieving of several months ago, talking about it with my therapist and my wonderful friend Kathy (who has two biological children, but amazingly *understands*), and just plain time have conspired to make me ready for adoption. No real regrets or second thoughts now—just a lot of impatience.

In the process of therapy I did a lot of thinking about what it all means. Why couldn't I get pregnant? Why is it almost an impossibility for so many women I know? It is *not* us—that I know emphatically. It is not something we did or didn't do. It is pure, random bad luck. Five years down the road, I know science will come up with the technology to get me pregnant. Ah well, bad timing as well as lousy cervical mucus and lazy ovaries are my fate. It just happened to me. So be it.

On the adoption front, I have been introduced to a local adoption counselor named Ellen Roseman. She has connections in the obstetrics community throughout the West, and she does a lot of outreach at high schools. She has a very good success rate and seems to have lots of birthmothers who contact her. I am particularly attracted to her service because she works very closely with both the adoptive couple and with the birthmother, counseling and maintaining contact with all concerned parties long after the adoption is complete. That sounds good to me. I don't think adoption is what happens the day the couple brings the baby home; it is, hopefully, a lifelong process. And I don't believe the myth that birthmothers forget . . . or should forget. They remember and need to know that they did the right thing. They deserve respect and attention. So, here's hoping something good will come out of working with Ellen.

Well, a blond shiksa from Philadelphia and an observant Jew: the mind reels. Details, please!

Wishing you time to write again soon.

Barbara

SEPTEMBER 21, 1985

Barbara,

My monthly week of treatment is now over, so I can return to my other life—my "other life" being the one that has nothing to do with infertility. This week was particularly difficult—five ultrasounds, two shots of the hormone HCG [human chorionic gonadotropin], three inseminations, a fight with the insurance company, and a scheduling nightmare between doctor and work. Now of course, the hardest part—I wait and wait and wait . . .

One would think that a female physician would be more sensitive to a working woman's needs, but it's not so. I have been told in essence that if I can't make the appointment, "hundreds of other women can"! I really hate the hold they have on me. If this were my dentist, dry cleaner, or grocery store, I'd take my business elsewhere—but in this case, there is no "elsewhere." Ken, I'm afraid, is at the end of his emotional rope. He wants to be supportive and usually is, but when I fall apart, he gets very upset and launches into his "It isn't worth it" lecture. He wants me to stop treatment (at least temporarily), but I am not ready to stop yet. I worry that I will never be able to stop. Every time we do not succeed, I think "next month," and that is what keeps me going. In the most recent *Resolve* newsletter a woman wrote that she has been an infertility patient for *fifteen* years. I cannot imagine it, and yet . . .

How is your "waiting game" going? Any significant leads? I continue to read in the paper about baby-selling cons and scandals, and I continue to be appalled at the exploitation of someone's *need*. I am glad you are being so careful. The counselor you discovered sounds like a great resource. As always, I'm hoping for you.

You asked about my Jewish connection. Well, pre-Ken, I was madly in love with a Jewish man. The feeling was mutual, even though he truly suffered over the fact that I am a blonde, Waspy shiksa whose father happens to be a minister! He spent a great deal of time explaining to me that our relationship was possible genocide for his people, and well, naturally, I felt very badly about that. To enhance the relationship, I decided to become the most Jewish Protestant ever, and I was quite a success. I kept kosher with him, learned a few key

Yiddish phrases, and attended a seder. Actually, it was a very enlightening year, but when the romance ended, so did everything else. Kind of a shame, as I am totally devoid of any specific ethnic roots.

Well, as usual, I've managed to ramble on forever. Receiving your letters and writing mine are wonderful therapy. How did I manage before? Know that I'm thinking of you.

Lynne

P.S. Ken and I will be in San Francisco in early March. Do you think we could meet? That's six months away—maybe by then . . .

SEPTEMBER 28, 1985

Dear Lynne,

The waiting game continues here too. We are busy writing our autobiographies, rewriting the "letter," and readying files and binders for Ellen Roseman. We wait to hear if we are ready to be added to her "active" clients list. We wait to hear if our lawyer has any new leads. We wait for the phone to ring. I am sick of waiting politely for the professionals—the doctors, lawyers, and counselors—to make something happen. We wait . . . and wait . . . you and I, for our babies. Doing *nothing* is the hardest thing.

I was standing at the kitchen sink, where I do some of my best thinking (and worst dishes), when it slowly dawned on me that the two men on the radio were talking about infertility. A highly "successful" infertility specialist was answering question after question from anxious woman after anxious woman. He was all gregarious confidence. It sounded as if there weren't an infertile woman in the Western world he couldn't cure. Never once did he or the program host broach the topic of failure, or of the interminable waiting, or of the emotional toll of infertility. When the doctor finally acknowledged human feelings are involved ("There is no question infertility is hard to bear, especially for men"), I slapped the dishrag into the soapy water (slapped soap in my eyes, too) and phoned the station. It was time to do *something*.

I started by telling the announcer I had a criticism to make. I said that, though I had no doubt that infertility is very hard on men, it is very hard—perhaps harder—on women. I reminded him that the vast majority of infertility patients are women and that for them—in contrast to men, for whom the diagnostic tests and surgeries usually occur over a relatively short period of time—it can seem, and can be, virtually endless: test after test and one invasive and scary procedure after another and month after month after month of drug treatment. Having no control over your body or your time can tear you—and your marriage—to ribbons.

Then the doctor asked what suggestions I would make to him. (The doctor was actually listening to me! Or so I thought.) I said I thought infertility patients, both men and women, need to hear the specialists acknowledge that they are not fully in control of the situation. They need to urge their patients to take some measure of control, whatever they can, over their infertility and their lives.

I knew what the next question would be. "And how have you taken control of *your* infertility?" I told him that I had taken control by choosing to end my emotional roller-coaster ride. After years of taking my temperature every morning, having one surgery or another, taking one drug or another, I said to myself one day that what I wanted most was a baby, more than a pregnancy. I told him it was hard, probably the hardest decision of my life, but that I am in so much better shape now. I said I am back to being myself and living my life again.

To which the good doctor responded by asking me if I was aware of a new treatment. In vitro fertilization. I thanked him for giving me the chance to talk and then said, "It is clear you haven't been listening to what I've been saying. I just hope your listeners were."

Then I bounced around the house like a complete idiot, shouting, "I'm a radio star! I'm a radio star!" When I'd calmed down a bit, I thought about some infertile woman somewhere in the Bay Area, standing over *her* kitchen sink, hopefully comforted in some measure by what I'd said.

Part of our work for Ellen Roseman these days is writing a more personal, more open letter directed to prospective birthmothers. I feel in my gut that this is a better approach. After all, open adoption is between birthparents and adoptive parents, not between doctors and adoptive parents. I am saddened at the wasted time writing, printing, and mailing thousands of copies of our first letter. It just means it will be that much longer until we find our child, and we aren't getting any younger. Lordy, WHY am I always the last one—to start a career, to meet a man, to get married, to become a mother? I have two friends my age who are already grandparents, for Pete's sake!!

Onward. This is a crazy trip we are on. Glad we have each other to share the ride with.

Love,
Barbara

P.S. I would love you to visit in March, babies or no babies.

OCTOBER 9, 1985

Barbara,

Congratulations on your radio debut—it sounds as though you were wonderful! We must continue to force the medical profession to understand and deal with the emotional impact of infertility. As for the comment from the caller about infertility being worse for men, I say bullshit! As usual, the infamous male ego is placed far above anything else and certainly above anything a woman could feel!

Since my last letter I have quite a bit of news—none of it good. First, my period arrived right on schedule. Six hundred dollars and sixty million sperm once again for naught. My single consolation is that it was on time, so I was spared any *significant* hoping. Amazing how desperate for good news I am. Anyway, as has become tradition, I screamed, cried, and was just generally miserable, and then I vowed to TRY AGAIN. Since then I've discovered "trying again" will be no easy task. You see, Ken has accepted a new job which will require relocation to Wisconsin. Despite the many advantages, there are equal disadvantages, and we have discussed both to death. For example, can

I continue treatment until we move? Doubtful, as Ken will go next month and probably commute until our house is sold. No Ken, no sperm, no insemination. Should I find a new doctor in Wisconsin? *Can* I find one? Also, what about my career, my profession? Clearly, there are no easy answers, but our decision was mutual, so I'll decide everything else as it occurs. In one of your letters you urged me to set a timeline for treatment, and though I know it's good advice, I simply couldn't do it before. Now maybe I will have to. I told Ken maybe that's why his job opportunity came when it did—to make us set deadlines. But he insists that my omen-seeking is a little too hocus-pocus for him, and besides, I'm getting kind of spooky. I think he's probably right. Anyway, on to yet another phase of my life which promises to be as complicated as the one I am leaving.

Any progress on your "search"? I truly understand your concern over the wasted time, and I cried when I read your comment about always being the "last one." You know, I keep reading letters in the *Resolve* newsletter that say things like—"Infertility was hard, but it was a learning experience" or "We've really grown since our adoption search began ten years ago" . . . and frankly I'm sick of it! I don't want to learn or grow anymore. I want a baby, *now*—and I want you to have one too!

Love,
Lynne

P.S. Can't wait for our meeting in March! We don't know when we'll be in San Francisco but anticipate early in the month.

OCTOBER 24, 1985

Dear Lynne,

It's all some sort of cosmic joke—I mean, our trying to become mothers and finding ourselves confronting one obstacle after another. Someone or something somewhere is getting a big chuckle watching our struggles and our determination not to quit. Like the Cowardly Lion in *The*

Wizard of Oz, you and I clench our fists and shout, "Let me at him, let me at him." The trouble is, we don't know who "he" is.

If the obstacle isn't the logistical complexities of artificial insemination when your husband is in another state, then it's having to write and rewrite an adoption letter to meet Ellen's standards—that being what I find myself spending hours on these days. Will any of this—solving logistical problems or dotting the i's and crossing the t's of a letter to a stranger—make any difference? Ask the Joker; don't ask me.

Unlike the Joker, I seem to be losing my sense of humor. I find it difficult to smile winningly as I jump through hoops for Ellen, as I go through this whole letter business ALL OVER AGAIN. (She says everyone has to pay their dues. Haven't I already paid, and with interest?) I know all the work and the search and the waiting and the disappointment must be dealt with—and I *will*—but, oh how I wish someone would just go out there and do it for me . . . and then present me with the beautiful baby that I know is waiting for me somewhere. Lord, I am weary of the endlessness of it all.

In a funny way, Lynne, I envy you having to deal with a problem (moving) that is so concrete, that has a beginning and a middle and an end. Right now I feel as if I will be preparing-to-start-to-begin-to-search FOR THE REST OF MY LIFE. (It would look interesting on my resume, don't you think: "Barbara Shulgold, schoolteacher and lifelong mother-wannabe".)

There, I feel better. Now back to those i's and t's. Keep me posted on the move. And for heaven's sake, be sure to let me know when you have a new address. I'd go nuts without a way to write to you and hear from you.

Love,
Barbara

Barbara,

So much has happened since my last letter, most of which is very good. I'm pleased to tell you that I have landed a great job in Wisconsin—I'll be in the labor relations department for a utility company, a position that offers many more opportunities than my current job. In addition, we sold our home after having it on the market only *two* days. It really felt like we were on a roll until last week—you guessed it; once again, infertility rears its ugly head. After yet another cycle with inseminations and everything else, my period was eight days late. A pregnancy test on Monday was "inconclusive." Inconclusive sounded wonderful until Wednesday, when I got my period, complete with cramps and a raging backache. On Friday, Ken and I met with my doctor for a final wrap-up consultation. We reviewed all the treatment I'd received, and she gave me a referral. As I prepared to leave the office for the last time, I totally fell apart. Somewhere in the midst of my hysteria, the bitchy receptionist I've dealt with forever also started to cry. She hugged me and said, "You really tried, Lynne." Needless to say, it was an emotional exit. I have now determined to take some time off from infertility treatment. So, my friend, I will not be pregnant for Christmas nor for our meeting in March—or for that matter, probably ever. But dammit, *someday, somehow* I will get my baby.

Did you see that miserable made-for-TV movie last week— "Whose Child Is This"—or something like that. It was about a couple who adopted a baby, and two years after the fact the birthmother tried to declare the adoption illegal in an attempt to get the child back. For your sanity, I hope you missed it.

What is the latest on your private adoption search? Have you sent your letters only to people in California or to people in other states as well? Are there certain states you won't send letters to because of legal restrictions on private adoption? Are the adoption laws of the state in which the birthparents reside those that are to be applied? Are there books on private adoption that would be helpful for me? Please send information—I think I will spend my respite time in research.

Well, must close. We leave for Wisconsin tomorrow. We will live in a hotel suite Monday through Friday and then return to Chicago on weekends. The escrow on our house does not close until January 6, so we will continue to get mail here, until then.

Take care—my hopes are always with you.

Love,
Lynne

THANKSGIVING, 1985

Dear Lynne, Eva and Bob (and Bill and Terry), Karen and Tammy,

Yes, I know: getting a xeroxed letter is the height of tacky, but when you hear our news, maybe you'll understand.

You guessed it: We've met a marvelous woman who has agreed to relinquish her baby to us. The due date is January 20! This time (in contrast to our painful experience with the woman in Texas last February) it feels real different, solid. It may be because we've met her—three times already. It may be because she's been seeing an adoption counselor who feels confident this is a *go*. And it may be because both of us intuitively feel good and right about all this. She actively interviewed us and came to see our home (particularly the nursery)—and that felt really good. The three of us share values (political activism, tolerance versus religious fundamentalism, and the importance of a good education were the three big issues for her) and communicate easily. So!

Also, her family (mother and two sisters) supports her decision. It was her mother, in fact, who suggested she relinquish. A supportive family is considered a significantly positive factor in whether or not adoptions work out.

Nancy is thirty, 5'4", 120 pounds, with light brown hair and hazel eyes. She's divorced, with a five-year-old son by her ex-husband, who is Jewish. She'd had a traumatic abortion in 1978 and swore she'd never have one again.

After getting her divorce last year, she moved to Florida, where she met and lived with the birthfather. The pregnancy split them up, so she returned to the Bay Area, where she and her son are now living in her mother's home.

She strikes us as very bright, forthright, strong—remarkably free of neuroses. She's a nonsmoker (no drugs either), moderate drinker, and athletic. Her family is clearly very well educated—all the birthmother stereotypes cease to function here!

The birthfather is in Florida still. He's 5'9", thirty-eight years old, with blond hair and blue eyes, and he's bright. Like Nancy, he's in telecommunication sales. He has very good health. We hope to learn more about him through the mail.

Right now we're heavily into negotiating about money (we're supporting her for four months), how it'll go in the hospital (Nancy says I can attend the birth—I'm thrilled!), relinquishment, and contact afterwards—all *very* delicate and emotional. It's taking up all our energy—writing this letter once is my limit these days. We are helped tremendously by Ellen Roseman, our adoption counselor, whose blunt speaking has helped us through some rough spots. She knows all of our fears and is smoothing the way for all of us. She says this looks like a very good one. I believe her.

Oh yes, how did we find her? After sending over 2,000 letters to virtually every state except California and waiting ten long, painful months, we contacted Ellen, now our counselor. She had us write an entirely new and different kind of letter. She wanted us to do 300 copies to send throughout California. But before we could do that, she gave us the names of fifteen doctors to send one to immediately. Voila! Three weeks later we got the call! Nancy said she read over 100 letters and chose ours because it spoke to her, and not a doctor. (I *love* Ellen Roseman!)

Exciting, scary, *expensive*. But we *are* going to be parents. (Even if this should fall through—highly unlikely—Ellen had two *other* leads for us the following week!)

Hold on, more news to follow. Keep your fingers crossed for us.

Much love,
Barbara

P.S. Lynne,

It means a lot to me to know that this news makes you happy (and
if you feel jealous, it's normal—for me, anyhow—as you know!)

All of this has been compounded by my having a uterine biopsy
the same week the phone call came (headline in my pessimistic head:
"Woman Tries/Fails to Get Pregnant—Gets Cancer Just As Baby Possibility Looms"). Turned out fine, but, as I'm still bleeding, I may need
a D&C—ugh!

How am I feeling? Thrilled (I deserve it), scared (if something
goes wrong?), and deeply thankful—for my health and my hope.

Wednesday we go for Nancy's doctor appointment and to hear
the fetal heart. OH!!

Books to read: *To Love and Let Go* (mandatory), *Co-operative
Adoption,* and *Dear Birthmother* (Corona Publishing Co., 1037 S. Al-
amo, San Antonio, TX 78210, $7.95). If adoption is your route to
motherhood, call Ellen Roseman.

Write soon. I want to hear about your job. A little package is on
its way (tee hee).

My best to you. Toast our hoped-for blessing, won't you?

Love,
Barbara

December 15, 1985

Dear Barbara,

I just received your letter and monumental news, and I cannot begin
to explain how I feel. Initially I cried—equal parts jealousy and self-
pity—but then, somehow, some way, I started to cry with joy, pure
simple joy, for you, my very special friend. You deserve this wonderful
baby and all the happiness it will bring. I know so well what went
before, and I am sincerely glad it is coming to an end.

The arrival of your baby gives me hope that I, too, will be a
mother someday. If you were here, I would hug you and scream and
jump up and down, but since you are not, know that I am thrilled!!!!

We are still commuting from Illinois to Wisconsin, but we just purchased a home and anticipate that escrow on the new home will close in early January. The house is beautiful—very contemporary, with one room perfect for a nursery (tell me *again* miracles can happen). I will send you the address as soon as I find out the zip code. I know the months ahead will be busy for you, but keep in touch when you can.

I am so *very* pleased for you.

Love,
Lynne

P.S. This Christmas photo of me, Ken, and his daughter, Annie, was Ken's idea. I'm sending it so you can have a good look at us, but I feel as though there should be a caption that asks, "Guess which person doesn't belong here?"

P.P.S. Please don't tell me that Annie "looks like she could be mine"; it is a comment I hear all too frequently.

DECEMBER 21, 1985

Dear Lynne,

The entire world seems propelled mindlessly toward Christmas. I am waiting for it to be *over,* so the calendar can move unimpeded toward January 20, Nancy's due date. C'mon, c'mon, let's go! Whatever happens when that baby arrives—good or bad I just want it to happen soon.

We have spent a lot of time with Nancy, both on the phone and in person. We went to her most recent doctor's appointment and heard the fetal heartbeat. I guess, never having been pregnant, I had never actually considered that the big stomachs women get have something in them. Does that ever sound dumb! I just hadn't thought what it would be like to have an almost-life moving and changing inside of me. I am thinking about it now, and I ache with the emptiness of my womb.

The heartbeat reminded me that there is something *real* inside there; someone, I mean—someone whose self-concept and self-esteem will be profoundly affected by Rich and me. I was quite moved and shaken. Then we went out to celebrate (hopefully not prematurely, excuse the pun) with the world's largest ice cream sundaes. Whoa, are we excited! We have also visited Nancy's home. It is her mother's, actually, a casually decorated Mediterranean overlooking tennis courts in a nearby town. Nancy is staying there until after the birth. In the evenings a roaring fire is always going in the fireplace. It feels friendly and comfortable there; Nancy's mother particularly seems to like us.

In a weird way we are adding more than a baby to our family— or maybe Nancy is adding us to her family. It is oddly exciting to be a participant in such an innovative way to make a new family. I hope this works.

I like visiting with them, although I do find myself trying very, very hard to please. The other evening I helped Molly, Nancy's sister, bring in bags of groceries and was embarrassed to find myself thinking, "Maybe doing this will make Molly like me."

Ellen repeatedly urges us to bring up all the sticky topics now: naming the baby, future contact, etc. Of course, I agree with her that all the delicate matters need to be discussed, but I am also acutely aware of how painful it is for Nancy . . . and scary for me. I discussed future contact with Nancy as I drove her home from the hospital tour. She made some quick comment about hearing from us once a year as she pulled herself out of the car. As to names, that was harder for me than her. I have had names chosen since I was seven and had never told anyone, except Rich. Being secretive about names is the only superstition I have; no one else will know them until after the baby is born. I won't even tell you, but I did get up my courage to tell Nancy and her mother. They liked them both. Such approval feels like a magic signal at this point.

Lynne, I have felt such despair, such hopelessness for so long, that it is particularly sweet to wake up each morning *anticipating* the day, rather than dreading it. It is sweet to watch (impatiently) as time moves closer to the due date, rather than hating each moment as it only makes me older and no closer to my dream. I tingle all the time. The only other time I have ever felt so alive was when I first fell in love.

It must be hard to read all this happiness. I don't know if I could have tolerated receiving such a letter just a few months ago. I don't know how I could have written you without causing any pain. I considered just not writing this letter; but that would be breaking our promise of an honest, no-holds-barred correspondence. So, it is my hope that what seems to be the happy ending to my story will be a source of encouragement to you. This is a hard time for you, I am sure. I have had hard times too, but look at me now. Your time is coming. And I for one intend to be there screaming with joy when it does.

Love,
Barbara

DECEMBER 31, 1985

Barbara,

January 20 is circled in red in my date book in anticipation of your baby. I am hoping and praying that everything continues to go as planned. Please be sure that I am at the top of your list for announcements, pictures, and any other wonderful, silly, sentimental stuff you may wish to send. Barbara, I am truly happy for *you,* but damn, I'm sad for me!

It is New Year's Eve morning and I am at my office. There is no one else here today, but I needed a place to go. Another year has slipped away, and rather than being excited about the future, I find I am very depressed over the past. I really thought I was dried up and cried out, but I guess not. Hang on, while I wallow a few minutes.

Okay, I'm back, feeling no better but sufficiently blown, wiped, and dabbed.

We moved into our new home on December 27 and are now gearing up for a series of contractors who will paint, paper, and repair. Even with all that needs to be done, the house is beautiful. There are lots of skylights, with glass and beams. I've been told there is also a great deck off the kitchen, but three feet of snow has totally obscured any view of it. The neighborhood is nice and, of course, filled with children. One rather aggressive six-year-old rang the doorbell yesterday and said, "Ya got any kids?" When I told him no, he walked off in disgust saying, "No fair." My sentiments exactly! "Concentrate on your fabulous new job," Ken keeps saying, and I'm trying to. Last Tuesday I lunched with the vice-president of my area and then Thursday was assigned my own hard hat for a coffee break with the "boys" in the plant. In truth, the latter was more enjoyable. At the end of the month I'll be attending a conference in New York City (and I've convinced Ken to join me there for a few days), and several more interesting trips are planned in the future. So, yes, I like my work; but it is not, nor will it ever be, a replacement for having a child.

On the adoption scene—appointments have been set for initial interviews at several agencies. At least on the phone, *no one is at all optimistic.* I've done nothing yet in regard to private adoption. Please tell me how to contact the counselor you used, the costs involved, and any other pertinent details.

Well, I best gather up my gear and go home now—Annie is arriving at noon and will stay for the remainder of the week. Funny, but despite the hassles, this little girl has become a comfort to me. I know she isn't my daughter, but she confides in me, wants to hang around with me, and I know truly cares for me. From my time with Annie, I realize the work involved in child rearing, but oh the rewards! How very fortunate you are to be embarking on all of this. I will hold my breath until the 20th and think of you, as always, often.

Love,
Lynne

P.S. I received your house-warming gift—thank you, the potholders are already hanging in my new kitchen!

JANUARY 6, 1986

Dear Lynne,

I know, I know—you just got a letter from me, but I am so moved by your New Year's Eve letter, I just had to write right away. Our letters certainly move each other—your tears moved me to tears.

This may sound screwy, but I'm glad you wallowed. Last year was the shits for you, and what a good way to *end* it. Try to think of those tears as being cathartic, leaving 1985's pain behind. Onward to *resolution*! (If *I* can do it, so can you. And you *will*. I believe that.)

Adoption: I've sent you a list of books, yes? Read them! And try to get Ken to. (My method: "Hey Rich, listen to this . . . " An hour later I'd see him reading the book.)

What about these golden cradle–type agencies—the ones that take only a limited number of couples each year? Expensive, yes ($10,000 to $12,000), but if you can afford it, you're guaranteed a baby before the year is over.

The open-adoption route we took is much less expensive ($3,000 to $4,000) but involves a *lot* of your energy and time. I really want to talk to you about it in March (if I'm conscious from lack of sleep).

Ellen Roseman: sharp, intuitive, and she'll make you work. But talking to her (and writing to *me*—hint hint) will take away the pain and loneliness.

If she happens to be in the Bay Area when you're here, you should make a point to go see her. Make no mistake: it's lots of work. But, Lynne, this infertility work has your baby at the end of it!

Your house sounds just *fantastic*! What's the setting? Send pictures (so *I* can eat *my* heart out).

And on your job: *Mazel tov*! I am genuinely impressed at your expertise and proud of you.

Yes, you will get silly baby pictures, etc., and always, my friendship.

Barbara

The card that Lynne had been eagerly awaiting finally arrived on
February 4th:

> *Miriam Leah Shulgold-Albert*
> *January 31, 1986*
> *5 pounds 9 ounces*
> *19 inches*
> *Rich and Barbara*

Six days later another card arrived:

> *February 7, 1986*
>
> *With great regret and sadness, we must inform you
> that our first child was removed from our home by
> the birthmother.*
> *Please allow us a week of private time to grieve.*
> *If you've sent cards or gifts, we will acknowl-
> edge them when we have our second child. We
> believe, since you are our friends, you will under-
> stand.*
>
> *Barbara & Rich*

You'll give me a big hug when I see you in March, yes? Cry for me,
Lynne.

FEBRUARY 10, 1986

Barbara,

There are simply no words.

I have cried for you. My insides are torn apart—my heart broken and the tears still won't stop. If I could, I would carry your grief for you, because you have had enough.

You are constantly in my thoughts and prayers. Write when you are ready.

Love,
Lynne

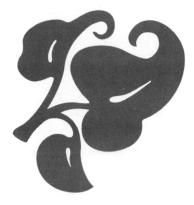

Homecoming

Dear Lynne,

It's taken two tall glasses of wine in the middle of the afternoon to help me get up the courage to write this to you. I came extremely close to calling you the other night, but figured you didn't need to hear my voice for the first time in a state of wild hysteria. Anyhow, you are the only person who is going to get this—all of this—in writing. If you feel the need, now is a good time for a glass of wine.

By now you have received our mourning note, which has apparently crossed with a note you sent me. I have not opened it and will not until we have a baby. There is just so much pain a body can take, and warm congratulations from you, after all we have been through together, would be too much.

Our precious baby was with us for five days before the birthmother changed her mind. Five days was just long enough for BOTH of us to realize that a new life is indeed as breathtakingly, achingly wonderful as we had dreamed. We fell in love, could not keep our eyes or hands off her, and even loved the exhaustion of the 3:00 A.M. feedings. She was an easy baby, which of course makes our pain harder to bear. She would quiet instantly when we held her, and we held and cuddled and loved her all the time. We took rolls of pictures (I am afraid I sent you one with the birth announcement). We called everyone and told everyone, and I took a child-rearing leave, and my class sent me congratulations—tinged with sadness, as they did not know I was leaving—and the faculty (also kept totally in the dark) called endlessly with congratulations and—well, you get the picture. The most beautiful week of our lives was followed by the worst. Everyone has been extraordinarily wonderful, as they always are when someone dies (and this is as close to a death as I can imagine). The women in my adoption group have been super: fixing us meals, holding our hands, notifying all our friends, offering country homes for a getaway—you name it. They were here when the baby was taken away, and they held me and cried with us. I am so grateful. TIME OUT FOR A GODDAM KLEENEX.

So, they say, this happens about 5 to 10 percent of the time, particularly when the mother has no family support system (Nancy had tons), when she doesn't bond with the adoptive parents (we spent hours and hours and hours with her), when she is young (Nancy is thirty), or when she has no children of her own (she has a son). Big deal statistics. I don't think she was conning us; I think she was just one of those people who are not introspective and do not genuinely know their own minds until it is too late. I feel betrayed, raped, empty, and enraged.

Part of me worries about you and Melissa, a woman in my school district who keeps approaching and avoiding the idea of adoption, saying, "I'll believe it works when I see you holding your baby." I fear this has set her back a few steps.

And YOU: I know how strange and risky and expensive everything I have been writing to you about these many months has sounded. I know how badly you want to give birth to your own baby, but think about adoption "just in case." I hope it makes a hell of a lot of difference to you to know that here, in the midst of this hellish pain, albeit numbed a bit by alcohol, I am far more certain than ever that I will NEVER NEVER give up my search for a baby. This pain is worth it: I will be a mother. So will you.

As to Rich: He underwent the most amazing transformation. At first he was so scared to care for her that he almost threw up. Then the nurse came to give us parenting lessons, told us we were doing just fine and were the kind of people who would make great parents, showed us a few tricks, and left. And from then on there was no stopping him. HE became the expert on diapering techniques, burping, poop analysis—you name it. I took dozens of photos (gone now) of him kissing and cuddling her and just touching her cheek. SHIT, he really went for her hook, line, and sinker.

The night they took her, I watched him cry for the first time in the nine years I have known him. And he wept and wept and wept. I have awakened in the middle of the night to hear him crying. The difference is now he says, "Now I understand what you have been fighting for all these years. I will not rest until we have another baby, and it must be a newborn: they are nature's greatest creation." Well, I coulda told him. But, better late than never.

So, what now? Well, as the book title goes: first you cry. I am crying a lot, sleeping a lot, watching a lot of TV, and having a little too much wine. Also, ignoring the telephone and letting the machine take the condolence messages. Can't take it. I am retreating for a week, going back to my therapist who got me through the infertility crisis (I went to see her the morning after, and she cried more than I did; I was the one screaming—really screaming—in rage). I don't think I will be able to go back and face the class and the hundreds of kids at my school who know me and will ask what happened to my baby and the faculty . . . so, I am not going back. It may be a mistake, but I am going to look for temporary work *away* from children: working in a little store, or as a secretary or something. I need a break.

Needless to add, this is probably the worst time financially for me not to be working. The adoption cost us $3,500, and we just don't have an equivalent sum to start again. Our wonderful lawyer is beginning a campaign to try to get the money back, but since Nancy doesn't really have money or a job, I am hoping a guilt trip or two on her mother (a college professor, for God's sake) will get her to reimburse us. I will stop at nothing to get the money back, including taking her to court, although I am as yet unsure if the agreement was legally binding. But my rage is real, and I have no intention of just giving up. THAT is impossible.

Ellen Roseman, upon whom all our hopes are now placed, assures us we are at the top of her list. I would not be surprised if we have a baby in three months. She is marvelous. She has had all sorts of former clients who have gone through the same heartbreak call us. All but one have babies now and were so comforting. Sometimes I think I would be a basket case were it not for the Resolve/adoption group/ Ellen Roseman networks.

You will be here in early March, yes? Spending time with you in person has now become an important future event for me. I guess, friend, there will be time for the two of us to talk uninterrupted by a baby's squalls, dammit. I do look forward to it, believe me.

My therapist says she admires me for enduring what I have endured, says that she sees me as a strong woman and that I will survive. You know, even now I can see that she is right. But, dammit, I would like to be weak for a while, and I would like to be a mother.

I know, I feel, how you hurt for me, Lynne. And it is a comfort.

Love,
Barbara

FEBRUARY 17, 1986

Dear Friend,

For ten days now I have thought of you constantly—at work, at home, and in the middle of the night. Your loss felt like my own and, frankly, I didn't know if either of us could survive it. But your letter arrived Friday, and though it broke my heart to read the details, I know now that we will be okay. Take some time to be weak, but never forget that deep down inside you *are* strong, so *very* strong . . .

You are absolutely right to try to get your money back, and I would not rest until I did. It is hard to feel empathy for Nancy, given all the time you spent with her prior to the birth of the baby. Do you think she understands that her change of mind has totally changed your lives? Like you, I am angry with her, and it feels good—damn good—to have *someone* to be angry at, rather than my old nameless, faceless, enemy—fate.

You floored me when you wondered how your experience might affect my feelings on adoption. Your capacity to care never ends. Well, it has affected me, but in a way you probably wouldn't expect. Ken was the one who handed me your February 7 postcard. He had gotten home early, picked up the mail, and was sitting at the kitchen table with tears in his eyes when I walked in. We talked about it and you and Rich constantly. Then your letter came and we talked more, and we have decided that if you can proceed after all of this, certainly we can begin. Now that probably doesn't sound very dramatic, but it is. You see, you were right—adoption always was a "just in case" with us, but no longer. In addition (to my utter disbelief), Ken is even considering a foreign-born child, which previously he had felt to be out of the question. Somehow in some way your experience got us over the hurdle. Yesterday Ken even explained our plans to his daughter.

There is so much more I want to say to you, but there will be time. You are alive and healthy and smart and intact—and so am I—and we will get what we want.

Love,
Lynne

P.S. The week before last I was in New York City on business and took an extra day to see the sights. Right after the Statue of Liberty and before Bloomingdale's I went to St. Patrick's Cathedral. I went on a whim, primarily because I am an architecture buff and the building is truly magnificent. I was totally unprepared for my reaction upon entering. Mass was in progress, incense was burning, and the largest organ I've every seen was being played. Being a wishy-washy Protestant at best, I have no idea what Catholic protocol is, but I noticed a variety of altars, each complete with its own marble statue and surrounded by candles. In the crowd (congregation?) was a woman who obviously knew the ropes—she was crossing herself and kneeling a lot and—well anyway, I quietly interrupted her crossing and kneeling and inquired about the statues and candles. She explained that each statue was a saint, and each saint has been specifically assigned to his or her own area of expertise—you know, Saint Francis and animals, etc. One need only make a "small donation" to light a candle beside the saint of one's choice and make a request. I must admit that I was totally intrigued by this, as Protestants have no such specialists. We simply must rely on God to prioritize, independently, the broken legs, brain tumors, and terminal diseases. Anyway, I circled the church looking for an appropriate saint for us. The Virgin Mary seemed an obvious choice, but she was getting a lot of traffic that day, and all of her candles were already lit. I almost stopped at a guy who does "lost causes," but that seemed so pessimistic and also too generic; but right next to him was Elizabeth. Elizabeth, though not the Patron Saint of Infertility, handles all the special requests of expectant mothers, and I decided that we fit there. I literally emptied my purse into the donation box and lit fifty candles—twenty-five for you and twenty-five for me. Previously dark Elizabeth was left in a blaze of glory. So, friend, the way I see it is that between my Protestantism, your Judaism and "Liz," we have it covered.

Dear, dear friend,

I have spent much of the last week wondering how I would ever find the words to express my feelings about your last letter. I don't think I can articulate to you or anyone else (and I have tried) just how much it meant to me.

Maybe I can start by saying that the letter has found a permanent place in my purse, so that I can read it when I need its comfort. Maybe I should admit that I have shared it with a few very select friends— something I have never done before with any of your letters, or anyone else's, for that matter. Maybe I should tell you that when Rich read it, the lump in his throat made it impossible for him to talk for several minutes. And I could tell you that my very fertile best friend could not stop raving about what an extraordinary gift it was. Or that my *new* friend Mary Ellen (more about her later) lunged for the Kleenex box as she read it and was astounded at the change wrought in Ken and the power of correspondence—pointing out to me that undoubt-edly I had changed through it as much as I see that you have . . . but, of course, it is harder to see change in myself.

Or perhaps I should tell you that now this Jew understands what the meaning of redemption is, because your letter has to no small measure redeemed the pain of my loss, has given it some meaning. Of course, I would rather have the baby and to hell with redemption; but since I cannot, I have felt tremendous strength and courage from your words.

I should tell you that your totally hilarious postscript caused me to cry and laugh simultaneously—no small feat, particularly at this point in my life.

Finally, I should tell you that I am so grateful, Lynne, so grateful that my letter to the *Resolve* newsletter caused you to write to me in the first place. Who could have known that we would affect each other's lives so profoundly . . . or become such good friends. Thank you.

Your wonderful Valentine's Day package was also a delight. I was too embarrassed to mention to anyone—including my husband—who asked what they could do to make this time easier for me that I wanted little things to open, little surprises that would remind me that I am still a woman and a feminine one (for some reason I have lost my womanly sense for the time being). I fantasized a silk robe or a scarf or candies or . . . and then in the midst of a driving rainstorm, when I felt imprisoned in more ways than one here in our flat, your package arrived—the candies, soap, and talcum, all in that pretty wicker basket. Perfect—I love it. I am trying to take your advice and am being gentle with myself. Right after gorging on all the yummy candies you sent, I went off for a hot tub and a massage. I pretended you and all the too many infertile women I know were there in the hot tub with me, and we had a good old cry and conversation together.

Mary Ellen is one of the several women who contacted me through Ellen, our adoption counselor. She suffered similar pain when her adopted baby was taken away from her. Mary Ellen and I have a lot in common, notably, that we are both currently unemployed and feeling a little lost. So we get together once a week. The idea originally was that we would make lunch for each other, but she has insisted that she make it each time, because she wisely sees that I do not have the energy for that yet. We hike and go birding together, but mostly we talk about the pain and dealing with our sense of loss and sense of outrage. I get a lot out of our visits, because she is "ahead" of me in this and constantly reassures me that what I am feeling is normal, that she went through a similar stage. What would we all do without each other in this business, eh?

Are you and Ken coming here in March? I recall that is when you said you would be coming. Please let me know as soon as possible what the dates are, as I am starting to look for some part-time work, and I want to arrange it so I am not working when you are here. Also, let me know what kinds of things you want to see, as I love to be a tour guide. Also, you will be pleased to know that Rich is an architecture buff, too; in fact, he used to lead walking tours of the neighborhoods. He would love to show you some of San Francisco's more interesting structures.

Will I go to Nancy's mother's office early next week and confront her with all the courage and assertiveness I can muster about helping us to get some of our money back? That is the question I have been wrestling with. Clearly, that is our only option left (we sent Nancy a letter via our lawyer two weeks ago but have not heard a thing), and

I am the only person who can do it. I am rebelling deep inside, though: Why must life add insult to injury here? Why can't I just be left alone for a while? Well, Rich is not the person to deal with that kind of confrontation, and our lawyer says that he feels he would definitely not help matters by doing it; and since Nancy's mother and I got along (or so I thought), there is really no other choice. The sooner I get it behind me, the sooner I can start to let all the painful feelings go and begin healing in earnest. I know I have every moral and ethical right on my side; I am just so afraid she will simply tell me to go to hell, and that it is not her problem. Well, then at least this particular struggle would be over, and I could find a job (at $5 an hour?!) to begin to recoup the expenses.

(Mail just came, including a bill for $155 from the pediatrician who saw the baby in the hospital. Ah, there is pain again.)

I know I am at the top of Ellen's list and at the top of our lawyer's list, and I KNOW THAT I WILL HAVE A BABY, but the question is, Will I have the strength to deal with all the unknowns and with a birthmother . . . oy vey. Mary Ellen reminds me that what she has done is become considerably more detached and self-protective. I think that is a good idea. I kind of feel emotionally dead anyhow. Mary Ellen got a call from what sounds like a fine birthmother last week, incidentally, and the baby is due in early May. So there is hope.

That's it. That's my energy for today. Write when you can, and especially let me know when and if you are coming out.

My love,
Barbara

MARCH 5, 1986

Barbara,

I received your letter and felt so good that I was able to help. It seems like such a small act in exchange for what you have given me. How do you thank someone appropriately for infusing you with the courage to proceed, after a decade of struggle? I guess the answer is you don't—you simply savor the strength and pass it along when someone else needs it. I am "relieved," which certainly must be halfway toward "resolved," and it is because of *you,* my special friend.

Since I last wrote, we have contacted an international adoption agency. We have read all of the literature, talked endlessly, and decided to adopt a Korean infant. The cost will be about $10,000—and though you warned me, I was shocked! A third is due upon application, another third when the social worker's home-study report is done, and the final third when we get our baby. I'm afraid Ken and I are typical yuppies—high salaries, lots and lots of things, and cash poor. We are, however, determined to put aside the needed funds and make formal application on May 1. To do this we must cancel our trip to San Francisco and, as you must know, I am *very* disappointed. We contemplated taking the trip and moving back the application date, but the thought of waiting even another month or two is unbearable at this point. I know that you share my disappointment, and I also know you will understand. The total waiting time until placement is estimated at about ten to eighteen months. It feels like forever, but again we will need the time to save the money. I am thrilled, scared, hopeful, and cautious, all at the same time. I've no idea what the ramifications will be for a foreign child raised by a blonde-haired, blue-eyed mother in Wisconsin, but it feels right for both Ken and me.

Enough on my plans. How are *you* doing? I am so pleased that you have found Mary Ellen and already developed an important friendship. Has she had more than one baby removed by a birthmother? Dear God, I cannot stand it! Lean on her, Barbara; you deserve the support. Regarding Nancy and her mother—do what feels right. As I wrote earlier, my first inclination would be to fight for what I consider justice, but only you can determine how much more pain you can bear. Morals and ethics be damned—sometimes it's just too exhausting, and that is a good enough reason to leave it alone, if you want to.

I know you're sad and tired and drained. Please feel *no* obligation to write, but remember I think of you every single day and am sending you courage and love.

Lynne

Dear Lynne and Ken,

Exactly thirteen months ago we got our first serious adoption "lead." It was only ten days after several of our friends had come over for a spaghetti feed and envelope-stuffing party to help us get our adoption search letters in the mail. Everyone—not the least of all, us—was amazed and quite ecstatic at how quickly the lead came through.

The next day I got a phone call from a friend, requesting I tape record for her the "Prairie Home Companion" that would be on the radio that night. "I am not going to be home tonight," she lied. She already knew that the show that evening would be focusing on adoption.

We listened to the program as we taped it. Tears ran down our cheeks as we heard the story of the Minnesota family waiting for the arrival of their Korean baby. It was as if the program was being aired in celebration of our (supposedly) good news. After the program was over, the phone rang off the hook with calls from friends who had heard the show. At the time it seemed an auspicious sign for the future.

The future still holds promise for us—of that I am sure. But, somehow, the tape seems to hold promise more for your future than ours. I don't know if you should listen to it now or wait until your child is about to arrive. It is a beautiful story, just as I know yours will be. Keep it as a token of my special joy at having had some small part in helping to bring your future family into reality.

My best wishes,
Barbara

MARCH 15, 1986

Dear Lynne,

Lots to report, most of it positive (well, maybe that is too strong a word . . . let's try "better"). But most important, I was thrilled once again when I read in your letter of March 5 the seriousness of your commitment to adopt. I have had some personal/political ambivalence about international adoption in the past but, like many of my adoption network friends, am beginning to consider it as a serious possibility for adoption number two. I just don't think I could go through the uncertainty of private adoption again. Even if everything ended up fine, I would never be able to let go of terrible fears during the whole process. We are committed emotionally and financially to finishing up this open adoption—but doing it again? I don't know.

Is the name of the international agency Holt? I have heard some good things about them. There is also an agency called OURS. I will look through my adoption file when I am through with this letter and see what I can find on the subject. Keep me posted on your progress.

I was not surprised to hear that you will not be coming out here, but of course I was disappointed. However, I get so much pleasure from your letters that it was not a terrible disappointment. Someday we will meet in person, maybe not until our kids are teenagers, but that would be fine! I certainly can understand your having to watch your pennies now as you save for the adoption.

Incidentally, I've heard that a lot of the golden cradle agencies (that is a generic term; I understand there are about a dozen of them throughout the country) charge between $10,000 and $12,000 for a healthy white infant. The other woman I used to write to via *Resolve* adopted in November through one of those agencies. The cost was $12,000 and the wait was six months. (They usually guarantee a baby within a year.) The disadvantage as I see it (besides the astronomical cost) is that you may not get a newborn (her son was almost three months when they got him). Of course, the adoption is final when you receive the child . . . which sounds pretty terrific from where I sit. If you want to learn more about the golden cradle agencies, I am sure my friend would be more than willing to help you. I'm enclosing her address.

You asked about Mary Ellen. No, she has not had more than one baby removed from her home, although the one she *did* lose, she had breastfed. She'd gotten herself a lactation counselor through La Leche League and had spent hours each day for weeks before the baby's birth massaging her breasts and using an electric breast pump. Heartbreaking. You should know that I have never heard of someone losing two babies. Ellen Roseman has found her a simply super birthmother who is due in early May. I watch Mary Ellen closely, because someday I will be in her position, and I am curious how she is handling the anxiety the second time. She says she feels a bit aloof from it all, and she talks a lot about the idea that the adoption may not work. All of that makes sense; she is being highly self-protective.

Mail just came. Today I got a note from a student in my class saying that she had heard we had lost our baby. I had tried to keep the news from the kids, but I knew that was essentially hopeless. It makes me feel badly to know the class knows; I can't quite explain why. I also know that now they are wondering why I have not come back to teach. Well, I just can't do anything about that.

As I was saying: Mary Ellen, I don't know what I would have done without her the day I finally got up my courage to go talk to Ann, Nancy's mother. Mary Ellen and I drove over to the college campus where Ann is a professor. I was *so* nervous. But that morning I had rehearsed with my therapist what I wanted to say, so I felt somewhat prepared. I was *not* prepared to walk into her office and see a picture of the baby at Nancy's breast. That started my tears, so I was not as articulate as I had hoped. But, what the hell! I laid everything on her: our grief, our loss of work time, and our enormous financial loss. Then, as I saw she was beginning to crumble into tears, I asked her to loan Nancy the money, so that we could begin to carry on with our lives.

She seemed to understand. She talked about how badly she felt for us, about how she had kept our pictures in the baby album (I didn't need to hear that). She said she thought we were wonderful people, that she thought we would be great parents, that she had been rooting for us. She also said that Nancy had grown increasingly depressed and, frankly, suicidal as the days went by after she had given us the baby. It is of no small comfort to me to be thus reassured that it was not a "scam." And I do feel better knowing that it was hard for Nancy.

She also said that she would talk to Nancy about giving her a loan so she could repay us as soon as possible. I went back this past week to see Ann again. She said that Nancy is very, very depressed about the way she screwed up our lives and her own. (I no longer feel I want to kick the shit out of her; I am almost sorry for her.) Nancy met with her two sisters and mother. According to Ann, the sisters will contribute as much as they can, and Ann—with Nancy cosigning—will take out a loan at the bank for the rest. She says we should receive the money in a couple of weeks. I am *so* proud of myself for confronting her in the first place; if not, none of this would have happened. I really do think we will get our money back. If we do, there is going to be quite a celebration around our house, let me tell you. If we don't, at least I got the family to acknowledge my pain. I think I am starting to heal.

I feel more free now to think about the future, specifically, what I will do with all the time remaining until we get our baby. Returning to teaching is emotionally out of the question. A serious, full-time job is not a possibility, because I don't know WHAT I want to do, besides teach. Plus, whatever I do would be temporary. I thought about temp secretarial work downtown, and lo and behold, there in the classifieds I found an ad for a part-time receptionist position with the Oceanic Society. Perfect: low stress, (low salary), good hours, great organization, and the location is unbelievable—their office is in an old army fort right on the San Francisco Bay; I mean right on it! I'll have one of the most beautiful views in the world: the whole city, the bay, and the Golden Gate Bridge and Marin County. I will try to send you a picture of it, if you will remind me (I have been enjoying taking pictures lately). The job is scheduled to end in September, which is great. The only hitch would be if I get a baby before September. But I am sure they could find someone to take my place.

I am thinking if I get that money back, I won't feel so poor. I have decided my salary is to be spent, not saved. And Rich agrees. I find myself starting to lust for things again. That's a good sign. I must be getting better . . . no small thanks to your loving and encouraging notes.

My best to you. Your letters are *wonderful* medicine. Thanks.

Love,
Barbara

MARCH 25, 1986

Dear Barbara,

Spring has arrived in southern Wisconsin. Today's temperature is a balmy sixty-two degrees, sweaters have replaced coats, and our lawn is finally visible to the naked eye. Yes, friend—spring is in the air, but I for one will step on the first damn crocus that gets in my way. Today is the morning after a major depression brought on by a variety of factors. You've been so pleased with my recent progress that I *almost* put off writing until this had passed—almost . . .

Some of my problems have a new twist, but at the root of all of them is the same old thing—*babies,* or rather, lack of same. Like you, I am burned out by my job. "Personnel management" is a euphemism for a daily dose of ten to fifteen problems or issues that require resolution. To reach resolution I must negotiate, wheel, deal, hand-hold, and ultimately just hope that the problems go away. The issues are trying, boring, exhausting, and typically just jive. Obvious solution: resign. Not-so-obvious response: I can't. To adopt a baby requires money, *my* money. Due to current circumstances, Ken's income is solely devoted to huge mortgage payments on a too-large house, child support, and assorted upper-class crap, i.e., Audi, housekeeper, and car phone. I don't know how all this happened! I could change jobs I suppose, but it is unlikely I could match my current salary, and that would mean an even longer period of saving. Anyway, I feel very sorry for myself. "It's all a means to an end," says Ken, but patience is not one of my virtues, and besides, it has been *ten* years. Same song, new verse—thank God there is you. I am so glad that you went to Nancy's mother. As always, I admire your courage and sheer guts. It sounds as though you will recover the money—no consolation for your loss, I know, but certainly the very least that you deserve.

My head is pounding from the cheap red wine I consumed, in quantity, last night—so I'd better doze for now.

Keep writing—keep hoping.

Love,
Lynne

P.S. Someone once told me that all calves are born in the spring, and it seems to me most babies must be, too. Suddenly all pregnant women are on the street or jostling their huge stomachs next to me in grocery stores or movie theatres. There was a time when this caused me a great deal of agony, but interestingly enough, I *am* over that.

APRIL 8, 1986

Dear Lynne,

We got the money back. Aha, you think, she must feel great. Well, I sure *thought* I would. Of course, I am relieved; but getting the baby ba (The preceding is a Freudian slip. I'll leave it in. It makes my point.) . . . What I meant to write was, getting the money back means that there is no longer hope of getting the baby back . . . a secret fantasy I could admit to no one—not you, not even myself. I didn't realize I felt that way till I held the check in my hand and burst into tears. I could see my baby's face again. I talked to her, told her goodbye, and kind of fell apart for a day. Then I went out and bought a bunch of pretty things that I didn't need. They weren't a baby, but they filled the hole, if only a little.

That was quite a day. A couple of hours after the mail, we got a phone call from Rich's dad telling us that his mother has cancer. It is in the gallbladder and has spread to the lymph nodes, but we do not know the site of origin yet. So, now it is my turn to hold Rich up. Being a grown-up is such fun! He is very nervous and quite frustrated being so far from his parents' home in Los Angeles. I suspect in the months to come he will be flying down a great deal. His family, unlike mine, is very unemotional and superrational. They are dealing with this in that fashion. It is very strange. I mean we are talking DEATH here. I am not particularly close to his mom; we have zero in common, except Rich. Mostly what I am feeling now is *scared*—not only for her but also for me: I think about my own health and aging. I guess, Lynne, it's because time is continuing to move inexorably, and I am still treading water, trying to reach my goal, and getting older! I guess what I am feeling is that I am dying. I would give a lot right now to be one of those who believe everything happens for a reason, but I'm not: I believe lives are largely governed by pure random luck. Nothing to do but keep on keeping on. Sometimes I am filled with cold panic.

That's not all that happened that day, either. Ellen called from Phoenix to ask us how we felt about adopting twin boys . . . already born! They were a week old, and the teenage mother was definitely going to give them up. We talked about it for a long time and decided against it (though I did consider splitting them with you!). Twins are a tremendous amount of work. It was hard, but neither one of us regrets it. I told Ellen that I trusted she understood we were not being snooty, that we wanted to take more control this time. She was very understanding. It is clear to me that she considers us for every lead she gets, and that is an immense comfort. By the way, do you know there have been *five* leads already?

Something should happen soon. Though, to be honest, I am extremely ambivalent about a new adoption prospect: I want it to happen because I am so panicked about my age, but I dread like hell the idea of going through all that stress again. No matter how hard we try, we will be paranoid next time. I just want a baby, dammit. Come on, universe, give me a break!

Two couples I know—one is in my adoption group, and the other is Mary Ellen and her husband—are expecting babies in the next three weeks. I am happy for Robin, who had two stillbirths and made us dinner the night after our baby was taken, and for Mary Ellen, who has been invaluable in the last month. But Lordy, I am so jealous I want to scream. You know, I have never felt jealous of adoptive parents before. Plus, since I have a terrible time around newborns, it means I will either not be able to see these friends for a while (i.e., until I have my own baby), or I will feel pain seeing them with their children. BLEAGGH.

Your letter surprised me. I am constantly relearning the fact that the style in which people live does not necessarily reflect the amount of money they have in the bank.

But, if you will forgive my presumptuousness for a moment: If a baby means so much to you, what do you need a fancy car for? Couldn't you sell it and buy a Toyota or something, as a means of raising cash? Couldn't you guys do your own cleaning? (We do it every other weekend; I am learning to ignore dust . . . figure it is good practice for parenthood and its realities.) None of my business, of course, but when you think of all the things that have gotten in the way of our shared goal—doctors, our dumb bodies, for example— money at least is something you can do something about.

A little voice in the back of my head is saying, Shut up, Barbara. But in the continued spirit of honesty, I have to say I got angry at Ken. Why does it have to be *your* money? If he wants a child, why can't he sacrifice his lifestyle . . . (if only for a while), too? Arggh, I feel like I am stepping out of line here.

You say your job involves "negotiating, wheeling, dealing, hand-holding . . ." so you must be pretty good at all that. Maybe you . . . OH STOP IT, BARBARA.

I am really sorry that you too are burned out at your job. Funny isn't it, about service professionals invariably ending up burned out?

Just reread your letter. You know, I think the reason your letter made me angry about your financial situation and Ken is that it reads as if *you* are angry at him. Or is this my imagination? I am not going to write like this anymore . . . feel like I am meddling.

I am running out of energy but would like to share one of my latest fantasies with you: We meet at a resort in Colorado and just sit and talk and walk and talk and eat and giggle and drink and cry and forget for a while the burdens of our frustrations. Nice, eh?

Thank you for the postcard. The "Union Maid" on the front of the card looks at me from my bedroom mirror. Each morning I return the look and I flex my biceps along with her. WE CAN DO IT.

Love,
Barbara

P.S. Before you step on the "first damn crocus" you see, as you wrote re your frustration with the arrival of spring, a story: I had a relationship years ago with a man who lived in northern Alberta. Of course, it was primarily a pen-pal relationship. One spring I wrote that it was sixty-eight degrees and I was writing in the backyard. He wrote back that it was forty degrees below zero, and he was holding on till the first crocus arrived. I wrote that they must be very pretty—I'd never seen one; what did they look like when they flew by? A couple of weeks later I got an envelope from him. Inside he had written only one line: "Here, idiot, this is a crocus." Out fell one beautifully pressed flower. I grow a pot of them every spring to remind myself of all the beauty I have never seen (I still have never seen one come up out of the snow *au naturel*).

APRIL 18, 1986

Barbara,

I have just returned from a week-long seminar at the University of Michigan. Topic: emerging labor issues as a result of diversification. Reaction: yawn. Still, the time away gave me the opportunity to think of a number of issues that I am anxious to share with you. So make yourself a cup of tea, settle into a comfortable chair, and prepare yourself for a long one . . .

First—I received your letter, complete with financial analysis and (contrary to what you may have anticipated) was not the least bit offended. Since you already know the state of my cervical mucus, I feel we have long since crossed the boundaries of what might be considered "too personal." Anyway, everything you said was true, and I am pleased to announce that the first meeting of the Sipiora Budget Review Committee was held last night. Be assured that I will think of you each time I drop to my knees and scrub a toilet. Changing will be tough—but these days everything is.

You also said in your letter that you sensed I was angry at Ken and, in retrospect, you were right—I was, and sometimes still am. Though he is very supportive, I often feel as though he doesn't care as much about all of this as I do. I believe that he would do anything to make me happy, but I don't believe that is an appropriate reason for him to want to adopt a baby. He insists that that is *not* the reason, but I am still not sure. To date, I have called the agencies, made the contacts, set the appointments, etc. Once initiated, he eagerly participates—but I *always* initiate! I can't help wondering if his more low-key attitude is connected to the fact that he already has a child. In the past you have written that you feel you have "short-changed" Rich because of your infertility, and from my experience in my previous marriage, I understand that completely. But my current situation is equally difficult. Ken, *my* husband, *my* best friend, participated in a pregnancy, experienced a birth, reaped the benefits of a child—all without me. Ken tells me his first marriage was loveless, but he and his ex-wife still shared something that I know nothing about. Frequently my hurt turns to anger and an accompanying resentment, and though I do try to control it, I am not always successful. Typical second-marriage blues made worse with the infertility factor. For the fifty millionth time—*why me?*

Regarding my job, I am frustrated, but managing. Lately I have decided that while the previous generation forced women into the "housewife/mother" role, our generation has forced women into a "career" role. Reviewing my own experiences, I see now that I too did what was expected for a college-educated woman; a high-profile job was mandatory to my image. So many of my career-oriented friends regard my baby lament as absolutely archaic and question my commitment to feminism. This is not fair. I certainly don't believe *all* women should be mothers—only me! A feminist book on health issues I read recently described infertility treatment as "invasive procedures by the male-dominated medical profession." The underlying message was that such procedures should be avoided at any cost. Over and over I read articles which assert that a woman is no less complete without a baby—so why do I feel that I am? Your thoughts on the subject would be appreciated.

I am glad you got your money back; small consolation, I know, but it does allow you to go on with your plans. I too harbored a little fantasy that maybe *somehow, some way* your baby would be returned— I'm sorry that it didn't happen. I do understand. Five leads sound promising, and knowing you are at the top of Ellen's list has got to provide some comfort. We are meeting again this Saturday with Lutheran Social Services, an open-adoption agency, regarding formal application. In addition, my brother, a high school teacher in Albuquerque, will begin networking for us with his many social service contacts. I am closing no doors. All of this has got to pay off, but the waiting, always waiting, is unbearable. It looks as though you and I will celebrate our second Mother's Day together without children, but dammit, there will *not* be a third!

You have *also* become one of my best friends—I wanted to write that letters ago, but considering the fact that we have never met, I wasn't sure how you would react to it. You have saved my sanity a hundred times and given me something no one else has been able to—understanding.

Love,
Lynne

APRIL 28, 1986

Dear Lynne,

I love it! I just can't believe that I helped found the Sipiora Budget Committee. You are doing wonderful things for my ego! And, needless to add, when I dropped to my knees to clean our toilet today, I thought of you.

You asked my feelings on our generation forcing women into the career mode. I think somehow the point of the women's movement has been lost. Its original push was not "You're not a woman unless you have a job outside the home," nor was it ". . . and you must be a mother too." Classic double bind.

It's about options. A woman should have the right to choose the ways in which she can best contribute her expertise, whether at home or in the workplace, or both. Though I have to say I can't help feeling a great many women have unconsciously buckled under to social pressures, and the "choices" they make are not their true choices.

I honestly don't believe there is any (I repeat *any*) more important job on the planet than parenthood. I want to, I intend to, do it well.

Mother's Day is coming. I went to every card store I could find and asked if they sold an irreverent card for the holiday. You should have seen the funny looks I got! So, in lieu of the card I can't find for you, consider the above, as well as my congratulations to you *and* to me for knowing what we want, and who we are, and for our determination to make this our last Mother's Day not being mothers.

(Incidentally, your friends who think your desire for motherhood is archaic will feel a little differently when they get closer to midnight on their biological clocks. Mark my words!)

I am rushing off to the woods to do some birding early on the morning of Mother's Day (Rich will be in L.A. visiting his mother, appropriately). I will go with our friends Myrna and Bernard, two people who know they never want to be parents. They do seem to understand how painful the day will be for me and have promised to keep me busy and distracted. We will be far away from civilization until it is time for me to get Rich at the airport. I know they will not even bring up the subject. I will be thinking of you hard, especially the moment you first wake up: that is always the hardest for me on days like that. I hope you are kept busy . . . or keep yourself busy by writing to me.

Keep toughing it out . . . with me.

Love,
Barbara

P.S. How is your adoption search going? I thought you were going to try to adopt a Korean infant, and then in your last letter you mentioned you were meeting with Lutheran Social Services, an open-adoption agency. What's up?

Dear Lynne,

Caught myself recently writing you a letter in my head. It made me realize how important it is for me to feel I am not alone with my feelings and frustrations . . . and reinforced how very alone I frequently feel. Events lately have made me feel more isolated than ever.

Gary, the man up the street, chatting with me on the steps and—as usual—complaining that they are on the short end with money (with their maid and their BMW). "It really got bad last year when we bought the baby." Did he mean it, or was it a Freudian slip? Either way, I wanted to slug him.

. . . Robin, the woman in my adoption group whom I am closest to, calling to say that everything went wonderfully in Denver, and that she and her husband were home with their new son, Eric. She has been invaluable all these months. Like you, she has an irreverent and biting sense of humor. I sent her a present, called with my best wishes, and listened interestedly to her story, and God knows I wish her the best. If anyone deserves a baby, it is those two. Nevertheless, I feel deserted.

Unable to resist, I introduced myself to a couple in a restaurant with an obviously adopted child. (They were white and the child Filipino.) Turns out they have been married for twenty years, never intending to have children. They were living in Manila, high on the hog in that God-forsaken city, with three servants and a fat paycheck from Bank of America. The wife went with some of the other B of A wives to give out presents at the local orphanage at Christmas. A little nine-month-old crawled over to her, grabbed hold of her skirt, and wouldn't let go. A month later all the legalities were complete, and the boy was theirs. "Go to Manila, live there for a while, and you can have any child you want," they advised. I wanted to puke on their dinner.

Shelley, part of my network of women who had babies taken away, met me for lunch to share pictures of her new son. She more than deserves it: a complete hysterectomy thanks to DES. She advised me to get more aggressive, to write a new letter with little stickers on it ("Birthmothers love stickers, I hear"). I have no heart for that, and she understood; it is just that she wants me to have my baby soon. I do too, but I find going through all that shit again almost too much.

A few days after that, she called me to say that her letter has gotten a lead and she wanted me to have it. What a dear! The birthmother, due in August, lives in Pottsdam, New York, about as far from San Francisco as you can get. I froze with fear. How can I deal with all that I have to deal with in an open adoption all the way across the country? There is no one there to "check her out" for us—to see that she is sincere, etc. I immediately felt myself wanting to run in the other direction. I don't want this to become serious. Can you imagine how much it would cost for Rich and me to fly to New York, rent a car, get a hotel, eat, etc.? Ellen called to say she has heard what Shelley has done and is very excited for me. Now I feel misunderstood even by her.

So you see why I find myself talking to you in my head a lot these days.

Oh yes, one more, Mary Ellen: her baby is due tomorrow. I haven't heard from her in over a month. Maybe the baby has already come and she feels uncomfortable calling me. Maybe she is tired of being around me and my frustration. Maybe . . . but what difference does it make? She is, or is about to become, a mother. And I am not, and I am *terrified* of the unavoidable risks I have to take to become one.

IF THERE IS A SECOND TIME FOR US, IT IS GOING TO BE AN INTERNATIONAL ADOPTION. I HAVE *HAD* IT.

The baby up the street is about to turn one. I remember the day Rich told me Jennifer was pregnant. I was still on the Pergonal merry-go-round. I was so blind with jealousy that I began to *scream* my rage. Rich turned up the stereo full blast so no one would hear me. We actually considered moving, but realized we just couldn't afford it. So here I am, watching the kid learn to walk and talk. I am becoming bitter.

And freaked out. My age: Maybe Nancy has messed us up so royally that it will become impossible for us to ever have a second child. How could I have the energy for a four-year-old when I am fifty? What am I doing with my life, and why am I letting it slip away?

Hmm, this letter is turning into a bitch session extraordinaire. I am perennially grateful for this correspondence, but especially now:

it is so valuable to know there is one place I can completely express myself, no matter how negative.

Love,
Barbara

MAY 9, 1986

Barbara,

I'm sitting on our deck watching the sun go down in streaks of red and yellow. The night is very quiet. Ken is away, and I wish you were here sharing my bottle of wine with me. Since that isn't possible, I'll just write and write and write—or pass out, whichever comes first . . .

Today is a real mixed bag. I spent most of it in an arbitration hearing for my company. It went well and I was feeling terrific afterwards, when a colleague said, "You were great, Lynne. I wish my wife was more like you. All she can do is have babies." Well, you can figure out the rest. Goodbye terrific—hello miserable, unfulfilled, infertile me! I managed to escape quickly and cried myself all the way home . . . "All she can do is have babies."

You asked about our adoption progress—well, there is *none*! An application with "down payment" has been submitted to Lutheran Social Services. They have told us they will conduct an interview in our home in early 1987, and placement will be a year after that. We will meet with another international agency on Thursday. If they can do anything more quickly, we will get our money back from Lutheran Social Services and give it to them. I have also contacted an attorney. He has asked for a resume-like letter, financial statements, and photos—all have been sent. So my limbo state continues as we attempt to cover all bases. I really thought the process of adoption would require more participation, but again it all comes back to waiting. My commitment never wavers, but my energy does. Every day makes me more angry and more tired. It is all just a big black hole of "maybe" with no end in sight. Well, as predicted, I am drunk, a fitting start to the Mother's Day countdown . . .

Saturday, May 10, 1986

Bad night, last night. I truly share your sense of loneliness and isolation. In preparation for tomorrow's dreaded day, I called my own mother this morning. After the usual small talk she started to cry, telling me that my pain over infertility is all her fault. She taught me to love babies, she said, and promised me, as a little girl, that someday I would have my own. Despite the fact that she was clearly distressed, I thoroughly reveled in her grief. I know that sounds awful, but I was comforted that someone could share my hurt—does that make sense? Well, must close for today—I'm "doing brunch" tomorrow for Ken's family and frankly glad of it. I will chop, grate, and dice myself into a frenzy and try very hard not to think.

Sunday, May 11, 1986

My asparagus soufflé fell en route to the dining-room table, which I recognized immediately as an omen for the rest of the day. And, of course, I was right. It poured rain, my stepdaughter neglected to send a card, and Ken walked on eggshells around me, hoping to avoid my now infamous "stares." Once our company had left, I re-read all of your letters in "celebration" of the Day. "It's really just another Sunday," you wrote last year at this time—but we were more optimistic then, or at least I was. Naturally, I thought of you and wished you well. Happy Mother's Day, Barbara!

Monday, May 12, 1986

You know, I have never been able to intellectualize my need for a child. Unlike you, I cannot even say, with any conviction, that I want to give something back to the world. My desire is based solely on the need to hold an infant in my arms, or a toddler on my lap, to experience unconditional love and to some extent a mutual dependency. Sappy sentimental shit, but absolutely overpowering.

Well, I will end this here. Writing to you got me through the weekend. Was Mary Ellen's baby born? Has she called? Are you still in touch with Ellen Roseman? Anxious to hear from you.

Love,

L.

MAY 24, 1986

Dear Lynne,

Well, I *thought* I was going to have some news for you this week . . . like a baby (newborn variety). But, no go. It has been an amazing and tiring and frustrating week. I just want to sit and watch the world go by and forget I ever wanted to be a mother.

First, a call from our lawyer that there is in the Bay Area a JEWISH birthmother (generally considered an impossibility). She is real, and her name is Carol. And she didn't choose us. We spent an hour and a half (and $100) talking to her counselor, telling her how wonderful we were and how serious I am about my Jewish heritage, etc. The birthmother was making a choice between us and another couple in Ellen Roseman's service. The other couple have the worst adoption story I have heard: the birthmother took the baby back after four months. They went to court and everything, but to no avail. My heart breaks for them. And secretly I was rooting for them. Their pain should be ended as quickly as possible. In any case, the birthmother did choose them for the most amazing reason: hair color. There aren't a lot of blond Jews, but she is one, and apparently so is the woman in the other couple. Sure wish I had known that in advance: I wouldn't have lost two nights' sleep, and we wouldn't have had to go through the interview and spend the money if someone had just had the sense to ask me on the phone if I am blond. OY.

Simultaneously, Ellen called about a fourteen-year-old birthmother about fifty miles north of here. The due date is ANY MINUTE! You should have seen the two of us that night: we were so frightened and *conflicted* that it took all the courage we had to call her. We talked with her mother, a real nice woman but not at all sophisticated, about what adoption would entail. The girl had been in false labor all day, and the baby had dropped. We were really shaken. In any case, it turned out that they told Ellen the birthfather is Caucasian, and then they told me he is Hispanic/Puerto Rican. He has fled back to Mexico. So we would never know, *and* we would never have any medical information about him. Too much for us: we politely backed out. Since then, of course, I have been dreaming of how beautiful that child would have been.

So in three days, we went from two leads to none. No, not true. There is a third one I haven't even mentioned to you. It doesn't excite me very much, I guess because the due date is a *long* way off. I don't think I can stand to wait till October. Add Lily in Indiana to the list.

We got her as a lead through our lawyer. I have spoken to her at length on the phone and just received a TEN-page letter from her. She says she has put us at the top of her list. She is worth cultivating. Haven't I gotten *hard* about all this?

She is thirty-seven (as was the Jewish birthmother, incidentally), with three children from eleven to twenty, and is divorced and working less than half-time as a nurse's aide. Anyhow, she seems to be a newly "born again" person, but not rigidly so. I told her I am Jewish and that we considered ourselves very moral people, though not church-going. That seemed to satisfy her.

She had volunteered for artificial insemination for the people in her church who were infertile but could never get pregnant that way. Then lo and behold she became pregnant by a man she had been seeing. They have had some disagreements and have drifted apart.

I don't know why, but I haven't heard from Mary Ellen in six weeks or more. It's probably because of the hysteria and anxiety that set in just before the baby is to be born. In any case, Ellen Roseman tells me that a son, Ian, was born last weekend. I sent Mary Ellen a note and a card. I hope we will be able to maintain our friendship, but we will just have to see. That means everyone that lost a baby has a baby . . . except us. Soon, right? The trouble is I really don't believe it anymore. I feel I will be in this limbo forever. (Can you see an eighty-three-year-old woman waiting by the phone for a call from Ellen Roseman?)

Do you think the day will ever come when we will exchange letters filled with the frustrations of being stuck at home with babies? Do you think we will ever write to each other about how our instincts pushing us toward motherhood were right? About how fulfilled we feel, how happy? I am feeling very pessimistic these days. Very.

It is so easy for both of us to lose sight of our strengths in the midst of all this exasperating waiting. I hope you are able to look at your coup in the arbitration hearing and exult about how smart and articulate and competent you are. I am proud to have such a talented friend, though not surprised.

What was the upshot of your meeting with the second international adoption agency? Was their timetable any faster? Early 1987 for the home study?! Oh, Lynne, I can't stand it! I really hope the other agency is faster. Please let me know. It looks like in either case you have a long wait ahead of you. Welcome to the club. Have you thought about how you will deal with it? I am getting very conscious of the time and sunshine and pleasures I am throwing out the window because I don't have a baby. I don't want you to do the same. Why have you not contacted any golden cradle agencies? Don't they cost about the same, and aren't they a lot faster?

I don't mean to leave you with the notion that I desperately want to be a mother for primarily "intellectual" reasons (giving something back to the world). That is my intellectualization of the primal urge I feel. Of course, what I really, deeply, primarily want is what you want: "to hold an infant in my arms, or a toddler on my lap, to experience unconditional love and to some extent a mutual dependency." It is *not* "sentimental shit"! It is what makes the world go round, and hurray for us for helping to keep it spinning!

Hope to hear from you again before too many more spins of this world . . . and hope the spins until then are better for you, and me.

My best to you, friend,
Barbara

MAY 29, 1986

Barbara,

As usual, so much to write about, but I will begin with the adoption update.

On May 15 I visited international agency number two. It is operated out of a storefront by a pair of married social workers. Chad and Lisel (can you stand it?) have remained untouched by time since 1968. Both had shoulder-length hair, wore lots of fringe, and pushed massive quantities of herbal tea during our discussion. They are legit (I checked them out beforehand) and nice (in a back-to-nature sort of way). Anyway, I think they can help. They can complete a home study and send it to our country of choice by September 1, 1986. Based on what they know about Ken and me, they highly recommend Chile. So I should be thrilled, right? Wrong! I'm going crazy with questions like—What the hell do I know about Chile (except that I prefer it without kidney beans . . .)? Should I really place my fate in the hands of two people who have a poster of Jimi Hendrix in their office? Do I blow all my cash on Chile, thereby eliminating all other options, should any others come along? Can I switch gears once *again* on who my child will ultimately be? (The transition from blonde-haired, blue-eyed infant to Korean toddler had effectively been accomplished, I think.) And, of course, there are many other questions. Ken and I will talk again tonight, and, if nothing else, proceed with the home study. But yes, you're right, I have joined the waiting club.

You asked about the "Golden Cradle" agencies. Well, I have talked to a few; however, inflation has hit the baby market, like everything else, and typical costs now hover above $20,000. We cannot pay that and save for my postbaby retirement, so it is not an alternative.

Your Lily lead sounds promising. Yes, October does feel a long way off, but what the hell, it's a date—which is much better than my never-never land.

Oh Barbara, I truly share your aging fears. Time moves so quickly in some respects. Still, I am thrilled to leave May and as always am pinning my hopes on June. . . .

Switching subjects—I can't believe you've not heard from Mary Ellen! Promise me when you have your baby, I won't lose you. I think about this frequently and it scares me—it really does.

Well, I must close—leaving for Boston on June 7 for a much-needed vacation. I'll have a chowder in your honor and write again when I return.

Love,

L.

MAY 31, 1986

Dear Lynne,

Your letter arrived just a few minutes ago, and I am sitting down immediately to respond. This is not an *official letter* because I have tons to do today, and more importantly, it is the four-month anniversary of the birth of Nancy's baby, and I am having a time of it—don't even have the will to talk to *you*.

But I do have a couple of important things to say, and I will wait till next weekend to write my official letter.

I am VERY uneasy about the social worker couple you met with. How carefully did you check them out? How long have they been in business? How many clients have they had? Can you talk to former clients? How many adoptions a year do they do? What is the average waiting time? Why Chile? I tend to mistrust big organizations— whether public nonprofits or corporations—but here I confess to being very worried about the small size of the couple's business. My friend Karen is in Brazil right now picking up her son and daughter through the Holt agency (which is a reputable, nationally known organization for foreign adoptions). I will spare you the details, but even that reputable, nationally known agency muffed up several times, causing her a lot of pain and extra waiting. That seems inevitable, dammit, but I just think there is less risk with a larger, more established agency than with a storefront operation. Please get all my questions answered satisfactorily, so I at least can sleep at night.

Secondly, you have no fear of my ever disappearing from your life . . . I, like you, am a fiercely loyal person. I look forward to years of correspondence about motherhood, written hurriedly between loads of laundry and trips to PTA meetings and whatever. Yes. This will happen.

My love and assurance of continued friendship NO MATTER WHAT!

Barbara

June 5, 1986

Barbara,

I think I told you in my last letter that I would write again when I returned from vacation—well, I haven't left yet.

An incident occurred this week that has totally thrown my emotional well-being up for grabs (again), and I need a second opinion (yours). It's a rather long story, but I'll spare you all the details and just get to the point. Quite by accident I have become friends with a woman who is a computer consultant in our office. We've lunched several times and have had many "professional" chats. As we became closer, I came out of the infertility closet, so to speak, and told her my story. She listened intently and then said, "You really must see my husband." Bottom line: her husband is a fertility specialist. I had no idea.

The following evening Ken and I met Kathy and her husband for a drink. I told him about all of my treatment, our adoption plans, etc., and he suggested we give medical intervention just "one more shot." We committed to nothing and said we'd think it over. Crazy as this sounds, I am furious that this has come up. I had put it behind me, was moving forward, and now all the old shit has been stirred up again! To date we've made no decisions, but your input would be appreciated. No doubt we will talk it to death over vacation. Vacation, incidentally, will be tough. Sunday to Wednesday we'll be in Boston (business for Ken), but Wednesday to Sunday we'll be in Ocean City, New Jersey, at my parent's summer home. This is a little resort town where my family has owned a summer home forever. Every June all of us meet there for a few days, and every June my brother and his wife bring a new baby. We will bring Annie, and everyone will tell me quietly on the side, "Aren't you lucky you *at least* have her" . . . Sounds like a good time, yes? Think of me.

Love,
L.

JUNE 6, 1986

Dear Lynne,

This is the official letter.

Welcome back from Boston—such a great city. The last time— also the only time—I was there was ten years ago to visit my cousin in Plymouth. Also a notable time because the week I returned, I met Rich. I've always been grateful for *leaving* Boston.

I'm not sure my quick note was coherent—I really dashed it off. But I know how wildly frustrating this adoption business can be, and it is a lot easier working with a "big-time" lawyer or counselor or agency. I would be a basket case right now if I didn't know I can count on Ellen's network—it is massive. And I want to spare you as much frustration as possible, though there will undoubtedly be lots, dammit.

I have really hit a wall. I think the realization that we are once again negotiating *in earnest* with a birthmother (Lily in Indiana) has brought out all my fears and astounding anger. I should have guessed that this would happen, but I didn't. I just fell apart this week: deep depression, back spasms, even a miserable hemorrhoid for the first time in years! And insomnia: something new in my life. Rich and I have been fighting like cats and dogs; he thinks I should be fine already, for Pete's sake, and said he is sick and tired of my feeling sorry for myself. Well, at least he said it at last, instead of walking around on the eggshells he shares with Ken from time to time, yes? We finally went to a counselor who helped us immensely. She explained that we were both acting consistently with our typically sexist upbringings: boys are told that they are responsible for solving problems, girls are told it is okay to feel and to ask for support—which the boys angrily misunderstand as a demand for active help, rather than an empathetic ear. (So we turn to pen pals for empathy, right?) I thought that was succinct and accurate as hell. We went out for pie and ice cream to celebrate. The air seems clearer now—helped considerably by the fact that I took today off and spent it in bed . . . amazing how much better that makes me feel, to just *give in* and get it out of my system.

I am scared. So scared that I have seriously considered just forgetting the whole thing . . . until Rich reminded me that I would become a bitter, mean-spirited, jealous woman. He is right. This is a classic approach-avoidance situation, and I have to go for it. He seems a bit more sensitized after the counseling and has agreed to take a more active role in the negotiations to come. That helps a little.

Today a note from Ellen about two other possibilities: a baby due in July in Tempe and another (due date not told) in Baytown . . . mere minutes from where our *first* birthmother lives in Texas. She was the one who changed her mind just a few weeks before her due date— which was the date you wrote me your first letter (helped me a lot later, knowing that *something* good happened to me on that day). Why do I feel like this is where I came in? . . .

I sent Mary Ellen a congratulatory card and then did, in fact, get a call from her, going on and on about the adoption scenes in the hospital, what it is like breastfeeding, etc. Jealous? YOU BET! She said she had been hysterical for weeks before the birth and that was why she hadn't written or called. I guess I understand. She said she will call again. I am kind of in a wait-and-see mode at the moment.

Onward. Write soon.

Love,
Barbara

JUNE 12, 1986

Dear Lynne,

Sitting in the Oakland airport, waiting to board my plane to L.A., I'm spending a few days with an old, dear friend and then joining Rich at his parents' home for Father's Day, which also happens to be his mother's birthday. I thought I'd better see his mom before she gets really ill. (She is down to seventy-nine pounds already . . . Rich has warned me to be ready for a shock.)

I'll be met at the airport by another infertile woman, who has a year-old daughter born by a surrogate mother. She's being sensitive, making sure I don't have to spend a lot of time with the baby.

I know this is also the same time you're with your family in New Jersey, and I am thinking of you.

I was overwhelmed by the letter you wrote in late February explaining the decision you and Ken had made to adopt. It is still in my wallet, read often and treasured. It eased so much of my pain; you'll never know what a gift you gave me.

I shared its sentiment and a few select phrases with friends but never shared this secret doubt I felt: I have experienced too much and read too much about infertility and its resolution to feel totally comfortable with your rather abrupt decision to give up trying to get pregnant and instead try to adopt.

I feel resolving infertility is a process. It takes thought and time and a hell of a lot of unconscious processing to let go of the dream of carrying your own biological child. It's important, *vitally* important, that you be thoroughly comfortable and positive about adoption as a choice before you become a mother—for your sake and also for the child's sake. (There seems to be a lot of evidence that psychological damage can be done to adoptees whose parents haven't resolved their infertility.)

(Time out for takeoff)

So although I suspect you have already made up your minds (if only unconsciously), I'll tell you my feeling. If the possibility of success with the new doctor is appealing at all, I think you should go for it. *You will either get pregnant, or it will help you get closer to resolution.*

I keep forgetting how much younger you are than I am. You have time on your side, and time burdens you with the titillating possibility of success ("Maybe this time . . . "). My biological time clock forced my hand, and I am grateful for that. It is *such* a fiercely hard decision to make. But making it, grieving it, finishing it (with the help of my supportive therapist, Deborah) is over for me. I think if it were over for you, you'd react as I did last year when the guy on the radio talk show asked me, "Why don't you try in vitro?": "Hey, listen, there is a limit and I've reached it."

You said the suggestion you give it one more shot made you

angry. Boy, I can dig that! What a bitch of an emotional roller coaster it can be. But, Lynne, this time it can be different for you; it can be something you're doing while waiting for your adopted baby. You'll be in a "can't lose" situation; you'll have less invested in it emotionally; and, though you will certainly end up with one child, you might end up with *two*!

Don't freak out. It's not as scary as it sounds.

One technique I've found very helpful in making decisions like this: Imagine yourself ten years down the road with an adopted child. Will you wonder if that "last shot" would have done the trick, or will you feel great that you didn't put yourself through it? Life is full of enough regrets; make sure your decision doesn't add another one.

Me, I'm a bit jealous of your options . . . though not your decision! You have years I never had. If you get pregnant, I'll feel a little jealous, but mostly ecstatic: any victory for an infertile woman is my victory, and deserved.

(Landing: "Clear skies and sixty-nine degrees in L.A., folks," says the captain. You should *see* the smog; it looks filthy. Glad I left this town . . . for a multitude of reasons. More later.)

Friday the thirteenth (uh oh). The old friend I'm visiting has gone to work, and I have all day to rest, read, and write.

Lily is getting very serious, and it's affecting me in strange ways. She *called* a couple of weeks ago wondering why she hadn't heard from us. (It took me ages to get up the courage to write. My letter must have arrived the next day.) She has definitely chosen us. The thought of going through it all again made me crazy. I began having crying jags and got so depressed I spent two days in bed watching soaps. I really exploded at Rich; I think he is *beginning* to recognize how angry I am at having to write all the letters, make all the phone calls.

I don't know how it will go. It's going to be expensive. She has no medical insurance, so the medical fee would be at least $2,500. She'd need $150 per week for six weeks of not working. Then there's *her* lawyer's fee, our lawyer's fee ($1,300 total probably). Two round-trip tickets to Louisville, car rental, motel for four or five days, three meals a day out, etc.—probably $5,000 total.

I feel particularly crass discussing all this in money terms. I feel vulnerable and resistant to taking risks. I'm starting to understand paranoia!

Needless to add, I am anxious to hear how your "New Joisey" time went, and *what's happening on the adoption front*?

Love,
Barbara

JUNE 19, 1986

Barbara,

Boston was wonderful—it was a business trip for Ken and a vacation for me, and we both thoroughly enjoyed it! I spent my days touring Beacon Hill, devouring seafood, and reading in the Common; who could ask for anything more?

From Boston we flew to Philadelphia (my birthplace), picked up Annie (who came in from Chicago), and drove to my parents' seashore house. Despite the fact that the place was overrun by an assortment of relatives and babies, that too was a good time.

Now we are back at home, back at work, and back to the business of baby hunting. Regarding the latter, we have decided *no more* fertility treatment. It was and is tempting, but the possibility of success does not compensate for reinitiating all of that old trauma. We also will not work with Mr. and Mrs. Flowerchild—they are reputable, their references do check, but I'm not comfortable with them. This leaves Lutheran Social Services, a Golden Cradle agency in Chicago (cost: $20,000), and the Independent Adoption Center in Santa Barbara. I found the center through a friend of my mother's, and over the phone, at least, they've been very optimistic. So, the beat goes on. I'm encouraged with your progress with Lily. October is just three months away—twelve weeks—a speck of time within the whole context of waiting. Will you travel to Indiana to get the baby? Are any of your other leads promising? Send details; I continue to learn from you.

Also, in the next few weeks I will have completed our birthmother letter/resume. Would you be willing to critique?

I'm thinking of you—'til July.

Love,
Lynne

JULY 4, 1986

Dear Lynne,

Believe it or not, here I am once again in the waiting room of the Oakland airport. Rich and I are waiting to catch a flight to L.A. This time we are going to see his father, who had a stroke last week. We spent a couple of tense, hysterical days waiting for the phone call telling us he had died, but to everyone's surprise and delight, he has made almost a complete recovery. We are exhausted, relieved. His mom, still very ill, is depressed, so we thought we'd visit and care for her and cheer up his dad.

It feels as if our letters have crossed. But if you've read my letter urging you to consider "finishing" with infertility treatments, and you still feel right about adopting (no regrets, right?), then I'm behind you all the way. Just be sure you are clear on that.

Things have been angry around here lately. I found I was angry at everyone: Ellen for telling me we keep getting turned down by birthmothers because I'm Jewish and we're "old." Who needs it? Angry at Larry (our lawyer) because he keeps urging me to contact Lily more often; at Lily for calling Larry to find out why she hasn't heard from us. I know I should be grateful to her for being such an active, committed birthmother, but I *hate* dealing with any of this. (Three couples are in the waiting area showing off new wee ones to grandparents. I'm wondering if Rich's parents will live long enough for us to make such a trip.) And angry at Rich for being so peripheral about all this. Once again I have to take the risks and the initiative.

So I pulled what as a kid I used to call a hissy. I refused to deal with any of it. In other words, I refused to be Superwoman. Larry and Rich said if someone didn't talk to Lily, we'd lose her. I agreed and said someone had better. So, Rich called her.

I felt liberated and finally able to commit myself to Lily, who is really very sweet, straightforward, and trusting. I know nothing significant has changed: I am still the leader in all this. But at least I got some help.

Lily lives sixty miles from Louisville in Indiana. She's a Mennonite (amazing!) and nurse's aide making $150 a week. The birthfather is forty-five, a hypnotherapist and has already signed off his rights. So much for teenage birthparents.

The due date is either mid-September or October 1. I'll have to stay very busy between now and then. I'm amazed at how much rage, resentment, really, there is in me. I just do not want to go through any of this again. I am glad Lily isn't around here. If we'd met, my hostility would undoubtedly have put her off.

You ask if there are other leads. At the moment no. I think now we would only consider leads for babies due after Lily's baby is born.

Please tell me more about the Independent Adoption Center in Santa Barbara. Is that a Golden Cradle agency too? There is an Independent Adoption Center near here. I'm wondering if they're connected. (The local one is not a G.C. agency, though.)

Yes, I do want to see a rough draft of your adoption letter. I have seen a zillion and could give you some feedback. Also, remind me to send you my friend Marcia's. The content is OK, but it's the graphics you should notice. As much as I hate to admit it, graphics are very important in catching the birthmother's eye. From what I know of you, you have a good visual sense (your Xmas gift and the lovely Crabtree and Evelyn basket), so you might enjoy those decisions. . . .

The plane's about to land, so I'll close now. Sorry this hasn't been as energetic as usual, but I feel real negative . . . mainly about this trip.

Hope *you* had a good holiday.

Love,
Barbara

Dear Barbara,

July—I can't believe it. I don't know about you, but for me the best thing about this month is that they will finally unveil that damn Statue of Liberty and let us all get on with our lives already.

Yes, Barbara, I'm a bit testy today and other than this letter, will communicate with no one. In truth, "testy" is a weak euphemism for furious, pissed off, or as my mother would say, in a raging snit. The focus of my anger is the state of Wisconsin and all of their inane laws regarding independent adoption. Yesterday Ken and I met with an attorney for three hours. I'll spare you all the dreary details and tell you only that should we identify an out-of-state birthmother and come to some agreement, the baby would have to reside in *foster care,* while awaiting the termination of Parental Rights. I feel that this provision will completely eliminate this option for us (also the Santa Barbara Independent Adoption Center), as I cannot see any birthmother agreeing to a double placement, when local parents could take the child from the hospital to their home. Why is there always another roadblock? It seems as though I no sooner get over one issue when another pops up. I'm frustrated and exhausted and—well, you know all the rest . . .

Though it does no good whatsoever, I keep falling back into the "why me?" routine. This morning's lead story in the paper was about a father convicted of raping his four-*month*-old baby! The horror and inequity made me (literally) ill.

Still working with LSS and hoping for a spot in their September home-study group. This group is put together for all people awaiting foreign-born children. The purpose is to provide cultural information and simply share common feelings. It is the first official step in the agency's adoption process. Should we get in, we could receive a child (eighteen months to two years old) from the Philippines in 1987. Hoping—but not hopeful.

Enough of my lousy news—I'm encouraged about your progress. Lily in Indiana sounds committed. Have you stayed in close touch? Why do I sense a lack of enthusiasm from you regarding her? Indiana is not all that far from me. Is there some way I can help? Let me know.

How was your trip to L.A.? I assume Rich's mother's illness made it difficult. Regarding your family—do you have brothers or sisters? You've never mentioned either that I recall, and you seem to be much more friend-oriented. My most wonderful friend, Sue, is coming up for the 4th of July weekend, and I'm really looking forward to her visit. She has no understanding whatsoever of this *big* piece of my world (infertility, adoption, etc.), but she listens and cries when I do and screams when I do—and never, never ever, tells me to just "cheer up."

Well, I better close for now. I'm at my office and so far today have managed three personal letters, two calls to LSS, one call to the attorney, and one call to Ken—job responsibilities, as usual, are at the bottom of my list.

Love,
Lynne

JULY 6, 1986

Dear Lynne,

Just got home to your letter after a tiring and stressful time in L.A.

I really am very tired but wanted to dash this off before the week starts and also to try to play catch-up with our letters, which continue to cross. So excuse me if I border on the incoherent.

I am feeling more up about Lily all the time, but "enthusiasm" is a word that just doesn't fit in our adoption world. We lost it along with our innocence. I do think this is the one that will work out. I just try my damndest to keep it on the back burner and carry on with my day-to-day life. Hard to do, but worth the effort. I have lost enough time already.

I rage and weep and gasp with you over the misfortune of your once again seeming to be chosen for "Why Me Queen of the Month." I had no idea Wisconsin was so backward about adoption. You have friends and family in Pennsylvania and Illinois. Is it impossible to do the adoption there? Also, I have heard of people who got themselves accredited as foster homes and "sort of" cared for the child, with the adoptive mother hanging out there. There must be a creative way around all this. IS YOUR LAWYER AN ADOPTION ATTORNEY? Maybe this is all hopeless, and you are glaring at this piece of paper and wishing I would just shut up. I don't know what else to say. I just can't believe what you say is the last word. I know Ellen has clients all over the country. I will have to ask her.

I can't give you much right now. I have given and given to two sick in-laws all weekend. . . . Did *not* need that, or the nurse caring for Rich's father who at the age of twenty-six (after four miscarriages) is going to adopt a baby she heard about in the hospital. It is due in January. No letters, no search, no waiting, no nothing. *GROWL!!!!* Time for me.

I look forward to your next letter and hope your time with Sue helped.

Your friend,
Barbara

JULY 18, 1986

Dear Barbara,

Some thoughts on your last letter. Regarding Lily: I know it's difficult to go through all of this stuff again, and I understand (completely) your need to hold back for fear of hurt; but Barbara, you mustn't let this woman get away! She's carrying *your* baby, and she wants (and frankly deserves) your consistent attention. Keep going—you're so very close now!

Today I am convinced that both you and I will be successful. Last night I reread many of your letters, and over and over again I was amazed at the innate sense of resiliency that we both share. . . . It's so trite to call yourself a "survivor" these days, but that's what *we* really are. Anyway, I'm proud of our strength and our tenacity, and I'm convinced we will be rewarded soon.

Not much has changed for me since our last letter. I am still (a) on the Filipino waiting list, (b) holding an application from the Chicago Golden Cradle and saving money, and (c) preparing for a mass mailing of our resume. The Santa Barbara center I told you about has been most helpful with the latter. My mailing, however, will have to be confined to Wisconsin. As I mentioned in my last letter, the state laws here make interstate adoptions very close to impossible.

In one of our crossed letters you asked if I had dealt with the infertility treatment issue—and the answer is yes. Trying again is not in my best interest right now. I knew this from the start, but I needed the time and courage to say no. So I've said it, and I'll not look back. Does that make sense?

It is ninety-seven degrees in Wisconsin today, and all predictions say it will continue for a week. Despite that, summer has been rather enjoyable here. Almost everyone has a boat of some type or another, and we've spent a lot of time lakeside. Tell me about San Francisco's attractions. I did visit your city once. It was a three-day stop after a two-week trip to Hawaii (honeymoon—first marriage). As I recall, a tour of Alcatraz was *the* highlight of my entire experience—which, I suppose, should have tipped me off right away that that relationship was doomed. That was eleven years ago. If I knew then what I know now—well, I'm glad I didn't.

Well, best wrap this up—off to Chicago for the weekend— picking up Annie, visiting friends, and brunching with family. I think I told you that Annie is now fully informed of our adoption plans and as a result now requests weekly progress reports. This I need.

As always, I'm thinking of you.

Love,
Lynne

July 26, 1986

Dear Lynne,

As usual, you are so right. I appreciate very much your gently urging me to pay attention to Lily. Yes, of course, she deserves it. And I needed to be reminded that all of this is and will continue to be very hard for her, probably harder than it is for me.

After I got all (or most) of my frustration out at Rich, and after he took responsibility for calling Lily, and after I expressed some of my frustration to you in my last letter, I felt a lot better. I have been a good girl. Lily and I have spoken on the phone once, and I send her a note each week with her support check. I am also going to send her daughters San Francisco T-shirts. She continues to write long letters, which I am keeping. She sent us the name, address, and phone number of the birthfather. She seems to think he won't object to hearing from us, so that is a tremendous relief. After I write to you, I will draft a letter to him. Rich and I want to go over it carefully, so we will probably not send the final copy for a week or so.

A lot has changed since I last wrote. Rich's dad called us last weekend, leaving a message (on our phone machine) which sounded extremely shaky. We called and, sure enough, Rich's mom has taken a turn for the worse. The doctor thinks it may be the final two weeks. Rich is down in L.A. now and may very well call me tonight to fly down. I am grieved that she probably will not live to see her only "baby" grandchild (her other grandchildren entered the family as young children). She would have loved it. So Rich is going to tell her about Lily (we have kept it a total secret from virtually everyone we know, certainly from our families) He has even brought down Lily's picture to show. Did I tell you we finally got a picture from her? She looks remarkably like me, but much prettier. Once I saw the picture, incidentally, and I could put a face together with the voice on the phone, I felt much more committed—bonded, if you will.

I have received your birthday package. But since I am spending my birthday weekend alone, I have decided not to open it until the official day . . . giving myself at least one treat in a birthday bereft of treats. Whatever it is, I thank you for your generosity. (You are a *very* generous person, you know.)

I am not the person to tell you about San Francisco's attractions; that is what Rich is good at. I can't tell you how many times I have fantasized taking you on a tour of my city—especially the architectural wonders, and there are so many. Rich has the language to describe them; I just have the aesthetic appreciation. It would be such fun to show you the craftsman-style homes of Berkeley, the best Victorians in the city, including ours, of course. It is a wonderful, breathtaking city. I am enclosing a few pictures of our house we had made from old slides. They are not very good but give you some idea of what our place is like.

It is not at all impossible that I may invite myself to your home to await the call from Indiana. That is just one of several ideas we have on saving plane fare. More if that becomes a more serious possibility. Can't think of anyone I would rather endure the final wait with.

Love,
Barbara

AUGUST 1, 1986

Barbara,

We're moving—yes, again! Boy wonder (a.k.a. Ken) has accepted an excellent new position with a national brokerage firm in (of all places) Kansas City, Missouri. Now before you begin to think I am totally oppressed and/or crazy out of my mind, you should know my vote was affirmative. K.C. is hardly the garden spot of the country, but compared to Wisconsin, it is *adoption* heaven! Our attorney has done a lot of research and tells us the laws are very favorable (compared to "impossible" here), and the foreign agencies have *no* waiting lists at all. Based on that, I said, "Let's go." Leaving Chicago was tough; this will not be. Anyway, the plan is for Ken to leave September 2. He will rent an apartment there for the interim. I will stay in Wisconsin until the house sells. My estimated departure: November 1. Once I arrive, I will not be pursuing my career. I've decided to go full-time into the baby search, and if that doesn't take eight hours a day, then the rest of the time I'll rest (bring on the bonbons). Anyway, I'm excited. Very.

I'm sorry you spent your birthday without Rich. What is the latest on his mother? Did he tell her about Lily, as planned?

Glad you're being a "good girl" and doing your part. I'm so happy/excited/jealous/scared/etc. for you. This does sound right though—hang in there, it won't be long now. I would *love* it if you would come to my house for the final wait—repeat *love it!!!* Let me know.

More soon.

Love,
L.

AUGUST 5, 1986

Dear Lynne,

I no sooner had sealed your thank-you note last week when the phone rang. It was Rich. "She just died," he said. I knew it would be soon, but somewhere in the back of my mind was the belief, the hope, that she would live to see . . . or at least know about the child. I was numb with grief, in worse shape than Rich sounded . . . though he was very busy dealing with the details and caring, nursing really, for his dad. I spent the afternoon listening to Mozart's Requiem and feeling very cold.

I flew down two days later and spent the weekend with his family. His dad is a supremely sweet man (I love him because Rich has all his better qualities) from the Midwest who has always lived by the don't-show-your-feelings ethic. It was so hard for him, particularly because as a result of his stroke, he seems to have lost his sense of balance—temporarily, we hope. He has to be held when he walks (even with his walker) or changes clothes or gets out of a chair. Very humiliating for such an independent sort. And, of course, all of that made his feeling of lack of control and loss so much harder to bear.

We hired a "homemaker" to care for him, and we did so, too. We cooked and cleaned and kept him company. I tried all my techniques to get him to talk about his time with his wife, to begin to grieve. Even bought him Judy Tatelbaum's *The Courage to Grieve*, the wonderful book that got me through my own recent grief. But he kept most of it in. It was a terrible strain for all of us, certainly mostly for him. They were married for forty-eight years, happily. It makes me want to grab Rich and hold on tight and never let go. Bittersweet— that's the word for life.

Saturday, the family (ten of us) went to Long Beach and took a boat a mile out to sea. We had all brought flowers—I brought one flower from every bush and tree in her garden—and we dropped them over the side as her ashes were put to their final rest. There was an eerie silence, then everyone began to cry. I saw Rich's dad alone and unable to move in his chair. I went over, held him, and told him to cry. And he did. It was "awful," that is, both dreadful and full of awe. We delude ourselves when we believe we are in control. "We are at the whim of the universe"; all we have is each other.

Rich brought Lily's picture down to L.A., but no one ever saw it. We intend to fly down every other weekend until the baby is born, because after that who knows how often we will be able to go. One of these days we will tell his dad, but right now I think it would be a source of additional grief, knowing how much his wife wanted a baby grandchild.

We returned home to find a letter from Lily. I am beginning to feel that this adoption is going to happen and, classically Shulgold, am starting to worry about birth defects (she did not have an amnio-centesis). Today I bought a couple of San Francisco T-shirts for the girls and a S.F. visor for Lily.

Did I tell you we had a long talk with Lily's doctor, who is very supportive of all this . . . and who has two adopted children himself?! He is definitely in our court.

I also wrote to all the airlines that fly to Louisville and explained our situation, i.e., that we cannot book in advance. I am hoping one of them will give us some kind of break. If not, one of the alternative plans is for me to book a mid-September flight (el cheapo) to Chicago and then bus or whatever to Wisconsin and stay with you until the baby is born. Rich would fly direct to Louisville, paying the full fare. From there we would drive to Albany, Indiana where Lily lives. I would love, repeat *love* to spend that time with you.

You're moving. I confess I am slack-jawed. I guess you haven't been in Wisconsin long enough for it to feel like home, but *moving:* that has to be one of my least favorite things to do. . . . You will be a little bit closer to me, and that's good. . . .

. . . But, are you sure you want to go there and not work? I think that sounds lonely and isolating . . . and inclined to make you obsess about adoption. The waiting in this business can just about do you in. Maybe you could volunteer, be a docent, take some classes—just so you could meet some neat women. I wonder if there is an adoption community there. Maybe a Resolve group?

The tiny closet-like room where I type my letters was not in any of the photos I sent you. . . . Our home is a wonderful, elegant place, but let me tell you the wainscoting and woodwork lose a bit of their charm when you have to dust them every week. I love this place, though; if it were a home instead of an apartment, we would probably stay here. Did I tell you it was once owned by Lotta Crabtree, a showgirl in the gold-rush era who is well known to San Franciscans? It is also the oldest building in our section of town; the upstairs was built in 1860. Then in 1880 our floor was built under it as it was raised. I hope very very much that sometime you can come out here and stay with us, and I will show you S.F.'s wonderful homes.

I must be doing well. Tomorrow is six months since the baby was taken. And yesterday when we got a new medical card in the mail for her, I didn't even cry. There is hope.

My love,
Barbara

P.S. I'm enclosing a good example of an adoption letter, written by my friend Melissa. I believe I have mentioned her previously. Her letters' graphics are what I want you to notice. Note how Melissa and her husband seem to *be* there on the page—great photo. Also, the frame around the picture really draws you to it.

P.P.S. . . . Would you consider using Ellen Roseman's adoption service? She has clients all over the country. I recommend her highly. She knows what she is doing. She will speed up the process for you. . . . Won't you consider giving her a call, or writing her? Think about it. Her card is enclosed.

AUGUST 11, 1986

Barbara,

I just received your letter with the news of Rich's mother. I have only experienced the death of my beloved grandmother, but that and the experience of infertility make me truly understand the pain of loss. I am so sorry. I am sure you are right—she would have loved your child. "Your child"—what wonderful words and how very soon you will be able to say them. I am so encouraged by all the positive communication with Lily. Surely even Shulgold the cynic must see that it is all falling into place. Yes? It is your turn, Barbara, and I am so convinced of that that there is no envy, only vicarious breath-holding, finger-crossing, anxiety-ridden joy! As we (note the "we") begin the countdown, please keep me informed. Even one line on a postcard would be appreciated if you can.

Since my last letter, the house has been placed for sale. Lots of traffic—no offers. Regardless, Ken leaves September 1. I have informed my office of the situation, and they accepted a rather open-ended resignation—which is just what I wanted.

Per your advice and my own conclusions—once in K.C. I will do *something.* Early retirement was a nice but short-lived fantasy. I just don't know what it will be. My skills and experience are in business, but I am so burned-out by the corporate environment.

No news on our adoption progress except that Ken has initiated the search in Kansas City. This may not seem particularly newsworthy, but it is. As I have written before, I have always been the one to do the research, make the calls, follow up. But this time (with nothing said by me) he started! More than ever I'm convinced this will happen for us too—some way, someday.

Thank you for the resume you sent. It was very impressive, though a bit slick, don't you think? My draft is ready and photo is to arrive Friday. I'll send you both.

Yes, I will call Ellen Roseman—soon.

Love,
Lynne

AUGUST 17, 1986

Dear Lynne,

"Surely even Shulgold the Cynic must see that it is all falling into place," you write. Well, yes, it does feel awfully good at the moment, but I persist in my cynical (?) belief that there is no one "place" for our lives to fall into; what I *am* uncynical about is the belief that if something should go wrong this time, I can survive it. I feel very much myself again; I think it has been years since I felt so in control, comfortable with my life. Of course, I am not in control of my fate, just of my ability to deal with what fate may deal me.

Wasn't even shaken—well, not *terribly* shaken—to hear that one couple from my Resolve group of years gone by had tried in vitro and succeeded. I just cannot believe that three years later, after all the changes and resolutions in my life, they were still at it. (There is, I confess, that small voice inside of me whispering, "You opted not to do in vitro. I wonder . . ." But the voice is quite small.)

We have heard nothing from the birthfather. I think I told you we wrote him a couple of weeks ago. Lily says he is not a writer, is almost always on the road. If we do not hear from him in another week, I am considering asking her to speak to him. Or maybe, just let it go. I would love to have his medical history, though.

I recently opened the note you wrote me, coincidentally, on the very day the baby was taken from us. In it you asked what was happening and to please let you know—a sweet note that made me cry . . . I really don't do that much anymore. Then in your most recent letter you asked me to please keep in touch, even a postcard, you wrote. I promise. In fact, if we fly through Chicago—or even if we don't, actually—I will try to call from the airport when we are changing planes. You will have to send me your phone number, though.

Your birthday and Lily's (and the due date) are in the same week. So last week, I took myself to the American Craft Council's craft fair. One of the finest in the country . . . is it ever in your area? Thought I would look to see if I could get something unique and wonderful (like our correspondence/friendship, no?) for you, and a gift for her. Instead I walked out with a most wonderful and special gift for *your* little one. So, friend, you had better go through with the adoption process, because I cannot wait to send it to you!

On that note, the book I wanted to send to you for your birthday is now out of print, and Rich refuses to part with his copy, so I am stumped. Stay tuned.

I am impressed—moved, in fact—with Ken's starting the adoption business in Kansas City. I don't know much about him, but clearly he has a sweet soul and loves his wife and his marriage. Sounds, in those respects at least, a lot like Rich.

I was sitting at a staff meeting at the Oceanic Society the other day when one of the women brought up the fact that a couple everyone but me knows is awaiting the birth of their privately adopted child. Discussion ensued on what a birthmother is, the risks involved, etc. I sat silently, bursting with feeling. Later, I found out that after the child is born, they are moving to Kansas City! So I thought I would try to get their names and maybe give them your address . . . might be someone to connect with there, since you have something important in common. If you don't want this connection, let me know.

I am VERY pleased that you are contacting Ellen. Let me know how that goes.

I also look forward to seeing your photo and letter.

Love,
Barbara

AUGUST 20, 1986

Barbara,

My special friend, understand that I am currently incapable of writing a long letter due to sheer emotional exhaustion. Still I want you to know our news:

1. Lutheran Social Services called. Due to the Aquino government, they now have several Filipino babies available for adoption in the immediate future.

2. They want to do a home study immediately—for placement in early 1987, providing we stay in Wisconsin.

3. We are staying in Wisconsin.

4. The house has been taken off the market. Ken has gone back to his old job, but I have not.

5. I will leave my job January 1 and then do some consultant work for the company, as needed.

6. Tonight is our first home-study meeting—I am scared to death!!!

7. My husband is the most wonderful man in the world.

More later—oh how I wish you were closer.

Love,
L.

SEPTEMBER 2, 1986

Dear Barbara,

As I know you've guessed, the last several weeks here have been unbelievable. As I told you in my quick note of August 20, just days after the house was put up for sale and we'd resigned from our respective jobs, Lutheran Social Services called saying we could be accepted into their Filipino program if we stayed in Wisconsin. It was, to me, the cruelest twist of fate so far, and I was devastated. As I broke my own record for the number of consecutive days in tears, Ken called everyone, everywhere. He was certain we could get around the residency requirement or hook up with a Kansas City affiliate of LSS, or postpone the move date, or well—you name it, he thought of it. When all was finally said and done, we realized there was only one way we could take advantage of the breakthrough with LSS—bypass the new job, the big bucks, and try to go back to the former employers. No one knows better than you how much I want a baby, but I couldn't ask Ken to do all that, I just couldn't . . . We agreed to think for a week and then decide our course of action on Friday night. On Thursday, Ken said he had already made his decision: "Family is most important—nothing else matters." He was able to get his job back, and he made the decision because he wanted to and because he knew I wouldn't harbor any guilt this way. Love does make all the difference in the world, and I get a little misty even now as I think of it all again.

Since that time we have started the study group required by LSS that prepares you for the adoption process. Tomorrow night is our third meeting and Thursday, our first home visit. We have been told to expect a boy—six to eighteen months of age—sometime in 1987. Ken is cautiously optimistic, but I have finally allowed myself to plan—names, furniture, clothing, preschools, etc. I am in deep, and I sincerely hope nothing goes wrong. Naturally, I will keep you posted.

Enough of my news—you must be wringing your hands and pacing now. Don't forget, you promised me a phone call. I'll be waiting.

Your birthday gift arrived, and as instructed, I've not opened it yet. My mother, who is admittedly biased, always told me that "all good things start in September." Maybe this September she will finally be proven right. I'll be thinking of you every step of the way.

Love,
Lynne

SEPTEMBER 2, 1986

Dear Lynne,

Have you been in my thoughts lately! I know just the sort of wild hysteria that has set in. Boy, do I know it. At last, you think, at last, I'm finally getting what I deserve. Well, dear dear friend, I hope so with all my heart. Wouldn't it be a wonderful end (beginning?) to our joint stories if we got our elusive babies at almost the same time? Wouldn't that be fantastic?

Well, hold on there. I am taking it upon myself to let a little air out of your bubble. (I certainly wouldn't pop that bubble.) I know, I know, you are thinking that I am now going to write from my cynical perspective, understandable after all I have been through. You're right. But I am also doing it to try to slow you down, to get your feet more firmly planted on the ground, to spare you as much pain and frustra-

tion as possible. I believe, I *believe* this will work out, for both of us
. . . eventually. In the meantime, remember the motto of all of us who
have (or who think we have) survived infertility wars: If anything can
go wrong, it will.

Especially when you are dealing not only with the myriad frustrations of an international adoption agency, but with the Philippine
government as well. Talk about a lumbering and inconsistent bureau-
cracy!! It will happen, but there are many surprises in store . . . and
many disappointments, too. I hope, when you send me your birth
announcement, that you can write, "Nyahh, Barbara, you were wrong
. . . so there!" I will dance with joy. Watching my friend Karen go
through her international adoption(s) was a lesson in frustration. She
stuck with it . . . just barely, and now has a sweet baby boy. But it
took months and months and months longer than she was led to
expect.

I hope you are not terribly angry with me for writing this. I am
doing it out of genuine love.

Your short, ecstatic, and exhausted note was a real thrill for me.
What a wonderful marriage you have! That Ken has gone as far up
the corporate ladder as he has and still has his priorities in order
speaks volumes both of the quality of his personality and the quality
of his love. You and I may have gotten screwed . . . figuratively . . .
in the pregnancy department, but we certainly ended up with a couple
of beauts in the husband department.

We are together in at least one other way: tomorrow Rich and I
have our home study. I can handle it. I can handle anything . . .
except losing a baby again. I think.

The escrow agreement has been signed by Lily and Rich and me.
Everything is going pretty well. The doctor has upped the due date
to the end of the month, as we all expected him to. "Waiting"—I
could write a book on the subject.

We received medical and personal histories on both the birthparents. It turns out that Lily smokes a half pack a day. I grabbed all
the information on smoking and pregnancy that Ellen had sent us and
read it immediately. Low birth weight is the most likely result, probably not brain damage. And, since the ultrasounds show it is a big
baby, I have decided not to worry. There is also some adult-onset
diabetes in her family, but that is the less serious kind and pretty easy

to control. Her children all had allergies which they outgrew. The birthfather: 6' 2", brown-haired. There is some kidney disease in his family, but I don't think that is inherited. . . . He is an only child.

Lily seems so passive much of the time, so compliant. I am frightened, Lynne. Rich has been forcing me to think about what I will do if this one falls through. The baby is due about the same time that my job ends. I would look for another temporary position or, worse still, do temporary secretarial work. I also think I might splurge a little and go visit friends . . . like you? I hope I don't come visit you now. I'd rather visit you later with a child in tow.

I feel good today. School starts tomorrow, and I will *not* be there. One good thing has come out of all of the pain of the last year: I know I can no longer teach. I think my next career should be motherhood. You too? You too!

Love,
Barbara

SEPTEMBER 8, 1986

Dear Barbara,

I received your letter Saturday, and (as usual) you have already anticipated my most recent phase in the adoption process. Euphoria has given way to a mounting impatience—now, already! Lutheran Social Services will simply not commit to a placement date and, when pressed, will only hint around at a "sort of sometime in 1987." The home study is, however, moving very quickly. Every Wednesday evening we meet with five other couples to watch child development films and read bad poetry on infertility (ode to a blocked fallopian tube . . .). Interestingly, all of the other couples have at least one child (either biological or adopted), which aggravates me to no end! What the hell are they doing there anyway? And, if they're going to come, shouldn't I at least be at the top of the list? These and many other questions go unasked as I continue my quest to be the social worker's favorite. Can you stand it—this reasonably well adjusted grown woman has been reduced to brownnosing—and, to make matters worse, Carolyn (the social worker) is a twenty-three-year old rookie!

"You're my very first group," she giggles, "and gosh and golly, I just know everything is going to turn out super!" I think I could deal with the terminally cute if she wasn't also completely disorganized. To date she's handed out four obsolete forms and lost three others that we'd already turned in. In any other situation I'd allow myself the luxury of an irate call to her supervisor, but this time my fate is in her hands. Does the craziness never end? In addition to all of this, last week we were given a laundry list of handicaps and were instructed to check those that we could deal with. It began with allergies and got increasingly severe. I know these are people we're talking about, but it became almost laughable as I attempted to talk Ken into a cleft palate or trade a hernia for an undescended testicle!!! On this subject— I would like your opinion. I really want a healthy child—doesn't everyone? But as adopters we're made to feel guilty about it. "If you really truly wanted a baby, you wouldn't mind that he was missing a leg"—well I would, and that in no way diminishes my desire for a child.

Well, I see that I have spent two and a half pages on me—your turn. Every day as I flip the pages on my calendar, I think of you and your soon-to-be-born baby. Though I can't stand the thought of anything going wrong, I think Rich is right to try to force you to think about the possibility. Throughout my life I have always tried to have a "Plan B," and though it never makes up for the loss of "A," it steadies you for awhile at least. You say Lily is being compliant; well, I would certainly prefer that to anything else she could be. Are you staying in daily contact now? I think I would be. Barbara, I know what an emotional risk this is for you, but I continue to believe it will all be worth it.

Tomorrow is my birthday. Another year . . .

Well, my friend, I better close for now. I've enclosed a copy of the photo we had taken for our resume.

As always, *thinking of you!*

Love,
Lynne

Dear Lynne,

A surprisingly drizzly Sunday morning, my favorite cantata program on the radio, a pot of Earl Grey, my elegant birthday robe, and time for a letter to you. Rich is in L.A. visiting and caring for his dad. I decided it was too close to the due date for both of us to be away from home. I have enjoyed the weekend alone, time for some serious thinking and cleaning and planning (I went a little nutso . . . *couldn't stand to wait any longer* . . . and bought a bumper for the crib and a comforter).

Ken's decision still reverberates in my brain. I have thought about it a lot. Surely it was done in part because the alternative would probably have been a lot of free-floating guilt in your home, but I believe along with you that it was primarily done out of genuine love for you . . . and a love for your *good* marriage. Which caused me to think: one of my worst characteristics is a tendency to look on the darker side of things. In reaching and reaching and yearning for the dream (a baby) I (you too?) seem to forget the special reality I have: a husband who loves me very much and who—like yours—has made many changes and sacrifices to show his love. I forget (you too?) how many MANY women I know have husbands who don't really respect them enough . . . enough to acknowledge their desires and to make changes, accommodations for them. I have always been Rich's equal, not "his woman"; I can't forget how special that is. Thanks, Ken, I needed that.

I can't say this enough: Hold on, Lynne, there are frustrations and disappointments ahead. You will end up with a baby (a son? Oy, am I excited!!) in the future. BUT it is farther away than you think. I don't want you to set yourself up for the disappointments. It's all bureaucratic bullshit, but between LSS and the Philippine government, there will be delays. Please try to live your life in the meantime (famous last words; do as I say, not as I do).

Is it impossible . . . financially impractical to go for private adoption at the same time? If nothing else, it would keep you busy, and a baby might come in sooner that way. AND have you considered adopting two babies/kids at the same time? I just know (do I know!) how excruciating the wait can be when all your eggs are in one basket.

Rich is still interested in considering international adoption for baby number two . . . if we feel we have the energy at forty-five to do it again . . . and if we are acceptable at that age. So, how much do you expect it to cost? You once said something like $10,000. I hope it's not that high. Details please.

Your study group sounds like another stroke of fate designed to make fun of or maybe test Lynne Sipiora. Once again you are surrounded by people who do not share your baby hunger. UNFAIR!! I know what that is like: I recently talked with Suzanne, the woman in my group who adopted first. She is "thinking" of starting the search for baby number two. "I'll get around to writing the letter one of these days; we're thinking of having a friend take our picture; I'm so busy with the baby, it is hard to find the time; etc., etc." When she and I started this process, she was more obsessed and depressed than I. Now it is like she is a member of another species. I can't imagine being so relaxed about it. Will I really be there someday?

AHEM, sermon number two for this letter: about the laundry list of handicaps. I feel very adamantly about that, so hold on while I vent my spleen. Look, you have been through it, you have paid your g.d. dues. The *least* you should get for all your grief is the option to have a healthy child. Had you given birth, you would have taken your own severely handicapped child—no question. But you didn't give birth. I feel strongly you should accept a child who is healthy by your definition, whatever that may be. Don't allow yourself to be guilt-tripped, Lynne. In fact, I feel if you are getting that message, it is because of incompetence/unprofessional behavior by someone at LSS . . . or you are doing it to yourself . . . because you aren't totally sure you deserve a healthy child. YOU DO!!

There, now I feel better.

We bought a new car. A Toyota Tercel wagon, beige. Just the sort of car middle-class women drive around with a baby in the back, right? Now, we *have* to adopt!

We received the most remarkable letter from Lily the other day.

She had called the Louisville airport and inquired about rental cars, rental baby seats, taxis, buses. Can you believe this woman? I mean, I was blown away. She is thinking about us! This is supposed to be an excellent sign (Nancy never so much as thanked us for the maternity top we gave her for Christmas). She also went over to the hospital to make sure everyone there knew we were to be treated as family and made sure it was okay for us to take pictures there. And she has arranged for her pastor to come and bless all of us. I am deeply touched and pleased as punch about it. I want that ritual, that blessing. And I am ecstatic that she is thinking about letting go. She also said she bought a blank journal to write to the baby before the birth. She tells me she writes poetry, so I have encouraged her to write some for the baby. So, please God, make this baby healthy. After being so cavalier on the last page telling *you* about your right to a healthy baby, now I find myself shaking in my boots, thinking about saying no. At this point I don't think I could actually say that.

I have been sitting here for a couple of minutes, staring at this page and wondering how many more letters you and I will exchange when both of us are without children. I even got a little misty there. Then I realized what is going on: If I were you, I would find it painful to receive frequent letters from a friend who had, and loved having, the one thing you do not have. Jealousy—my old nemesis. Is that how you feel? I would like you to write me, now, how you would like me to handle talking about the baby. Do you want me to be detailed, to send pictures, etc.? Or should I just be brief and go on to other things? Let me know.

If you get a child that is a year or so old, we may end up with kids the same age. What a great thought!!

Today I got a suitcase ready for the trip: modest/dull nice-girl clothes so I don't look like a city slicker in that small town, camera, baby clothes, diapers, bunting, car seat, film, Valium. The basics. The social worker thought we were nuts to agree to stay in Lily's house; I think she is right, but now it is too late. We have already agreed. She says it will be very emotional, and we won't have anywhere to go to be alone. The hospital is on Lily's block! We will be surrounded by her relatives, living with them, being judged by them . . . and nowhere to hide. Thus, the Valium.

Your home and work phone numbers are in my wallet. I will call. Cross your fingers.

Love,
Barbara

SEPTEMBER 27, 1986

Dear Lynne,

I was sure I'd get a letter from you today. Everything OK?

We are jittery wrecks, of course. It took three days to get up the courage to call Lily this week. I just *knew* it would be a nervous phone call. The baby has dropped, she's had a couple of sets of false labor pains, and the doctor says it could be any day. Took me an hour to calm down enough to realize I was not going to throw up for sure.

So, we spent all day cleaning the house (assuming we'll be too wiped out to do it for at least another month), making lists, packing, jumping every time the phone rang. Probably the baby will be born this week.

I'll call you on the way back home. So, assume up to ten days or so from today's date (9/27) you'll hear from me. Don't panic—it could be longer.

If none of this works out, I'll treat myself to calling you anyhow. So, one way or another, we should be talking soon.

Cross your fingers. Visualize positively and pray . . . to "St. Liz" for us.

Thinking of you. Wishing you were here.

Love,
Barbara

SEPTEMBER 29, 1986

Dear Barbara,

September 29 . . . since I have heard nothing from you yet, I will assume you are still awaiting "the call." I think of you constantly and have even taken to dreaming of you and Rich and cherubic-like babies dancing on clouds. Letter writing at a time like this is tough. I am fearful of saying anything that might jinx the deal. Crazy? Of course— but that's how I feel. So I'm going to change the subject, not because I don't care about whatever it is that is happening in your life but because I do, so very much.

Wednesday night is our last meeting of the adoption group— following that, we will simply receive calls from the social worker on a monthly basis. Naturally, I will keep in touch with the other couples, but I wonder if we'll be able to retain the camaraderie we have developed. Siblings, grandparents, and any other extended family members are invited to attend the last meeting. Annie will come with us, and I'm pleased we are able to get her involved. For the home study she was required to write something about her feelings on the subject, and with no coaching and/or assistance, she did. I've enclosed a copy. It truly touched me, especially when she pointed out it was in her "very best handwriting."

On the subject of "feel goods," I must tell you another story regarding my father-in-law. Dick is a kind of Archie Bunker type. He is a caring man, though, and because of that has done a lot of changing over the last ten years. I sometimes marvel at everything he has had to absorb: Ken's divorce and joint custody, and now infertility and an Asian grandchild. Still, he's done well, despite the fact that he frequently gets his information mixed up and always quotes the *Reader's Digest* as *the* source of vast knowledge. Anyway, last week he called me—it seems he'd been reading *Reader's Digest* again and had just read an article on infertility. "Lynne," he said, "I know it's none of my business, but I wanted to let you know there's a new procedure—just invented—that can be done in the doctor's office that can completely open up your *filipino* tubes." Bless him, I laughed for the rest of the day.

Well, my friend, it is nearing 7:30 A.M., and I must chug another cup of coffee and be on my way.

Everything will be OK.

Love,
Lynne

These are my thoughts of my future adopted baby brother.

First off, I would like it known that I personally think my father and stepmother are two of the best people on earth. Lynne is very understanding and also very down to earth. My father is the same. Dad really knows what is best to do. I believe they are doing the best thing. They are both caring and great people.

As you probably know, I am eleven years old. I have always wanted to have an Oriental brother. In fact, I have always wanted a baby brother. I'm really glad I will. I am looking forward to this greatly!

To conclude this letter, I would like to add a few more thoughts. Being a big sister-to-be, I would do only the best for the baby, which means a lot. I would help take care of him, take him to the park, read him books, and take him to the zoo.

I think the future little boy would fit in well with our family, country, and friends.

Ann Sipiora
September 14, 1986

MIRIAM ELENA* SHULGOLD-ALBERT

SEPTEMBER 29, 1986

7 LBS. 8 OZ.

RICH AND BARBARA

*To the Lynnes (Sipiora, who was there through it all, and Fingerman, who helped us to believe in open adoption), and the Ellens in our lives (Olshansky, who helped us Resolve our infertility, and Roseman, who was there for us when we needed her): This precious child, this fulfillment of our dream, is named in your honor for all you have done to help bring us to this happiness.

Of all the nerve, not being in your office when I called! In my excitement, I forgot to tell Ken, when I called from the Louisville airport: both birth-parents signed off all their rights. She's a keeper, Lynne!

My Love,
Barbara, a mother at last

Hope

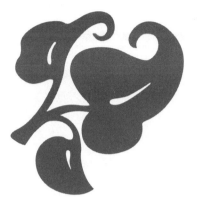

OCTOBER 1986

Beautiful, wonderful Miriam,

Ever since I heard about your impending arrival, I thought how very fortunate your mother was. Her precious baby—at last—the one we'd hoped and wished and waited for. But today, when I finally heard you were here, I realized how fortunate you are too—to be loved and cherished by my beautiful, wonderful friend.

All my love,
Lynne

OCTOBER 6, 1986

Dearest friend,

I'm sitting here on the floor watching Miriam stare at Ballet Bear as we've named her, and for the millionth time today I'm awash in tears. *Everything* makes me cry, certainly Miriam's gift from you, and your beautiful note. More than thank you.

It's all wondrous strange. She's ours (all rights signed off, by Lily and Robert), but we haven't bonded yet. Such a shock to get exactly what I've waited (forever?) for. It's beyond words.

And exhaustion: We are bone tired . . . living in fear we'll sleep through her cries and she'll starve. Unreasonable and natural new-parent hysteria.

Allow me a few weeks to gather my wits and emotion and strength and time. Then you'll hear from me. No way a baby is going to change our great friendship! In the meantime, keep writing and using me as a sounding board. I *love* hearing from you.

My thanks and gratitude.

Love,
Barbara

OCTOBER 12, 1986

Dear Barbara,

Like you, I can't stop crying. The pictures are wonderful—the joy so evident that my heart truly feels as though it will explode from emotion. I don't know how to tell you how much I care, but perhaps you can feel it even 3,000 miles away. I cried when I got the announcement and am touched by your choice of middle names. Then I cried over the thank-you note and totally lost it over the picture of you and Miriam in the rocker. Since this kid's been born, I haven't bothered with mascara but have invested heavily in Kleenex . . . and here I go again!

I want to call you, but I too need some time. My happiness for you is without hesitation, but I ache a little bit for me. However, don't you dare hold back any information because of that confession. I want to hear it all. What color are her eyes? Does she smell good? Is she as beautiful as she looks? Oh, how I would love to hold her myself!

Enjoy every minute, don't worry about writing. I will talk to you soon.

I love you, friend.

L.

OCTOBER 16, 1986

Dear Lynne,

It's one of those rare days when I think I am awake enough to try typing you a letter—the one I have been writing almost continuously in my head for a week now. (Rich did the middle-of-the-night feeding last night—bless him—and then went off to work this A.M., so I feel relatively rested . . . I doubt I will feel *really* rested for months, if then.)

The hardest thing, the thing I must write first, is that I have been thinking what I would be feeling if I were in your shoes. Mixed feelings, for sure, with an emphasis on jealousy, my old and perennial bugaboo. Everything has changed, but nothing has changed: I am still me, I still think the world of you and our life-sustaining correspondence. Everything has changed: I have reached my goal, I am a mother. (Reverse the order of the two preceding sentences, please.) Although I think for both of us at the beginning this correspondence was a means to help us get to our shared ends, I feel it has become more than that—I trust you do, too—and that our correspondence will continue as a valuable part of the unique process which is life.

As usual, I want to tell you everything; but to try to relay what went on in Albany, Indiana, alone would take pages. Rich has written it all down, in his vaguely journalistic style, calling it "The Miriam Chronicles," written to tell her about her beginnings. One of these days I will type it up, after we have jointly edited it; remind me to send you a copy.

Suffice it to say that it went as well as one would hope—so vastly different from our experience with Nancy that it is hard to believe. Lily is very strong and very courageous and incredibly trusting of us (although at the last minute at the urging of just about everyone in town she did ask us to sign an agreement about amount and frequency of future contact—letters and photos and visits. We suspected, rightly, that the agreement held no water legally but wanted to set *any* fears she might have at rest.) Her eleven-year-old daughter took a shine to me immediately (a schoolteacher—WOW) and shared secrets and schoolwork. Her sixteen-year-old was very resentful and clearly had to muster all her willpower to talk to us. I finally cornered her, burst into tears, and asked her to acknowledge me and what was happening and that we were not stealing her sister. It seemed to help; we cried on each other's shoulders for a while. Since then, she is slowly getting better, according to Lily.

Lily was gracious and trusting throughout. Her mind was and is made up. She knew it would cause her terrible suffering (it is) and she knew it was right and she knew she would have to grieve and begin to get better (she is). Talk about your unsung heroes!

The most moving part was in the hospital when she handed me the baby as the minister (to my surprise, with TWO adopted kids of his own from Korea—I told him about you) gave the most wonderful blessing, clearly written from the heart of his own experience of adoption. I can send you a copy of it, too, if you'd like. I am sending one to Ellen Roseman, as I bet there are lots of couples in her service who would love to use it.

On the plane, we remembered to open the letter Lily had handed us as we left with the baby. I don't think anyone on the plane, particularly the stewardesses cooing over the babe at that moment, could understand why the couple with the brand-new baby would both have tears streaming down their faces as the plane took off.

Miriam. Everything about her seems quite unreal to me, still. I check on her constantly, convinced I will go look in the cradle one time and she will be gone. The first congratulatory phone call came from Stacy Bischoff, the woman who had had the unfortunate role of taking Nancy's baby from us. When we heard her voice on the phone machine, both of us went white and my knees buckled. It took us a second to realize that she had nothing to do with this adoption. (In fact, she adopted a baby girl herself a month ago.) Rich put Miriam in a basket in the living room, after we had been home a few days, and then—as a joke—brought me in the bedroom where the cradle is and said, "See, she's gone already." I almost decked him.

She is new life. She is open to everything. Everything is a wonder in her eyes. She is a wonder to me, to us. We are mesmerized . . . but this is not the happy ending to the story, Lynne. This is the beginning of a new one.

And a strange beginning. Bonding . . . it takes time, and that can happen to anyone—biological or adoptive parent. And because of our history with Nancy, it will probably take us longer. Truth is, we both feel as if we are babysitting still. Probably by the time you get my next letter, all that will be history. But for now, some secret thoughts that shame me: I wonder if she will be pretty (would our biological child have been?) or smart (an article in today's paper on identical twins raised apart gives credence to the increasingly popular notion that IQ and skills are genetic . . . that environment plays a lesser part than previously thought). In other words, can I and will I love her "as if" she is my own . . . can I make her my own? From what every other adoptive mother I know has told me, my fears are common. You get past them, to the point where you cannot imagine the child as anyone else's; she or he was meant for you. I am not at that place yet. I am trusting that it will come. In the meantime, it is such a thrill, almost a physical one, to touch her and care for her and feel her cheek against mine. My favorite moment is when, in a feeding/rooting frenzy while being burped on my shoulder, she starts searching for the nipple and finds the thing nearest to her which most resembles the nipple: my nose. You haven't lived until you have had a fifteen-day-old infant suck your nose!!

I like being home. I literally haven't left the house in five days, just being a housewife (though who has the energy to cook or clean?). I admit to being a bit scared about taking her out: What if I run short of formula or have to change her in a supermarket or she starts to cry and I can't comfort her or . . . ? New-parent fears.

Rich is wonderful. He just loves being a daddy and seems almost more concerned with the state of her poop or the amount of formula she has taken (once again, he is graphing it!) than I am. I trust in nature's ability to care for itself. We are becoming boring already, talking only of her, getting so much from her. I realized the other night that we hardly cuddle anymore, compared to our usual rate: we are each cuddling with her instead.

It was all worth it.

Did you drink some Friexenet for us? We are still too tired to touch alcohol. Oh yes, sleep a few extra hours for me. You have no idea how incredibly seductive the thought of just lying down and sleeping can be . . .

Write soon.

Love,
Barbara

OCTOBER 21, 1986

Dear Barbara,

I received your most recent letter yesterday, and once again I see you've asked how I feel. Two years' worth of correspondence has served to convince me that you really care how I feel and typically understand how I feel. Given that, I'll answer. I feel lousy!

I am consumed with envy. I didn't think it would happen, but it has. Forgive me, Barbara, but I would much prefer to be the one who was writing the "be strong" notes. I knew, of course, that one of us would be first, and given the length of your wait, I was sure it would be you—but dear God, I wanted it to be me!

The arrival of Miriam makes my waiting harder to take. I don't know why. Ken says she is *our* symbol of hope, a flesh-and-blood reminder that it will be okay, but I'm afraid I've viewed her differently. Another baby that I do not have . . .

In addition to blatant jealousy, Miriam has made me rethink the entire foreign-born issue. I am having serious reservations—reinforced by two women who attended our last study-group meeting. Their Filipino children—billed as "healthy"—have been hospitalized for about 50 percent of their total placement time (one year). Asthma, respiratory problems, heart murmur, and some significant developmental delays due to malnutrition. Do I need this? Do I want this? If adoption is a second alternative to conception, is a foreign-born baby a third? These concerns are torturing me. Our original bee-bop social worker has been fired (surprise!), and a far more professional type has been assigned to us now. I have hinted at my fears with her, and she has recommended working concurrently with a Golden Cradle in Chicago. If somehow, some way we can get the money, we will do that. Still, regardless of the eventual source, waiting seems to be the name of the game . . . so what else is new?

October 22

Home from work with a miserable cold—period fifty-three days overdue, no doubt early menopause or maybe ovarian cancer—drinking tea, blowing my nose, and thoroughly enjoying my one-woman pity party. Was just about to write "wish you were here," but quickly remembered you no longer have a reason to wallow. Jealousy waning, but loneliness kicking in. Still, I'm curious about some things, though I'm sure it is still too early for you to answer, but—does the pain go away when you have your baby in your arms? Does the memory of the struggle to get her start to fade? Do pregnant women still piss you off? Can you remember how you felt before? Before must seem so long ago to you now . . .

Well, my friend, I'm going to drag my flu-ridden body back to bed, but before I do I must share with you what I think is a very funny story. A guest speaker at our adoption group told it, and I relay it because of your frequent mention of "lack of sleep," which, incidentally, I have not one bit of sympathy for . . . On that note—it seems a new adoptive mother was sitting in her home with her best friend when new baby begins to cry for the hundredth time that day. Said mother of child looks at friend and says, "I suppose you think I asked for it," to which friend replies, "Hell, honey, you begged for it!"

Much love,
Lynne

NOVEMBER 10, 1986

Dear Barbara,

I have not heard from you in awhile and assume it is because you are exhausted and/or any other associated rigors of motherhood. At least I hope that is the reason and *not* because my last letter hurt or offended. I must confess to being a little embarrassed by the jealousy I felt (let's be honest: *feel*), but to date our relationship has been built on honesty even when the honesty has gone beyond the parameters of "nice." Mixed up with my envy is a real sense of loneliness—surely now I am the only woman left in America without a baby. . . . Anyway, I feel sorry for me, and I don't give a damn if that's not admirable—it is how I feel. Your empathy is welcome and furthermore, solicited . . .

Last Friday night we hosted a party for our LSS adoption group. A very interesting combination of people with nothing in common except the adoption. Still, even in that group my need and desire seem stronger than the rest. At first the evening was a little awkward, but after several hours and several bottles, people started to open up. Much to my surprise, everyone seemed to share my concerns about foreign adoption, and (even more surprising) all agreed they would go the Golden Cradle route if they had the money. Based on that, I am further convinced that this is the best option available. Several months ago a friend suggested a Golden Cradle in Chicago—cost, $25,000. I spoke to their executive director, and he was very encouraging. My plan is to apply December 1 ($2,000 to register) and then "beg, borrow, and steal" until placement—at which time the balance is due. Ken is apprehensive, but a jar on our dresser labeled "Baby '87—FULL RETAIL" convinces me he, too, has come around. I have not called Ellen Roseman yet and am not sure that I will. It is becoming so difficult to juggle all the sources and information that I don't know if I can handle another one. I'll keep you posted.

My job here ends January 10; and, as you know, I'd planned to take the bonbon route, but that's no longer an alternative. Though my heart is really not in it, I do already have several pending opportunities.

Okay, enough of me and my plans—tell me about wonderful Miriam. Has she grown and/or changed? Have you found the courage yet to take her out? Has your family seen her? How is big Daddy taking it all? Is she pretty-sweet-good? Has she made you forget all that went before?

Your homecoming picture remains on my refrigerator, and I think of you daily.

Write when you can.

Love,
Lynne

November 14, 1986

Dear Lynne,

The Divine Ms. M looks like she may sleep for a while (I never can tell: sometimes it is for three minutes, sometimes it is for three hours), so I will try to answer your letters. This—and all other letters for the next eighteen years—may get interrupted and have to be done in bits and snatches.

First of all, you are right and wrong. Yes, I have not answered because I have had very few continuous minutes to myself . . . and those I do get, I use to sleep or do laundry. But, I have been avoiding answering you, as you hoped I hadn't done. I *knew* from about the third or fourth time we exchanged letters that it would come to this— that one of us, probably me, would get a baby first, and where would that leave the other one? And that this friendship would be severely tested by such an event. And that I didn't know what I would say when it happened. Well, it's happened, and I still don't know what to say. I have spent many of my (few) conscious moments figuring what I could say in response to your October 21 letter. I value our friendship and respect your need for honest expression too much to pretend, to ignore your jealousy, to shield you from what it is like to be a mother at last.

So, I guess the best I can do is say I wish it were otherwise right now. I wish we were both mothers right now. My considerable happiness would be easily doubled if that were so. Since it isn't, I hope you will get comfort and assurance from my letters and evidence that if it happened to me, it can happen to you, too. It will, Lynne, and until and *after* it does, I will be here for you.

Before I get to your two most recent letters, I would like to go back to one you wrote on September 29, and which was waiting for me when we got back from Indiana. Known as the Filipino Tubes letter, it ends: "Well, my friend, it is nearing 7:30 A.M., and I must chug another cup of coffee and be on my way. Everything will be okay." Amazing. Do you realize that Miriam was born at 7:33 A.M. your time, that very day? You wrote that letter as she was being born! I recently reread it and realized that; brought tears all over again.

On October 22 you wrote asking if the pain goes away, if pregnant women still piss me off. Let me tell you about the first meeting of my mothers' support group. I walked in firmly expecting to be walking out in a couple of hours filled with jealousy over the labor and delivery stories I would be hearing. What a surprise to discover that most of their stories sounded pretty yucky; I was not at all envious of all their pain and risks. Except for one woman—quite pretty, with a remarkably pretty baby: I thought her baby was the only one there that clearly looked like its mother. Was I wrong! It turned out she is an adoptive mother, too. She talked about sending out only 300 letters before getting *two* leads, one of which they turned down. Their whole time in the adoption biz was slightly over three months. I could've killed her. I was so pissed. I guess I've resolved my infertility issues, but not my feelings about all the frustration and grief we went through in the adoption process.

You don't let go of strong feelings easily—I guess that is what I am learning. They fade slowly . . . just as love and bonding grow slowly. Slowly, surely, we are falling hopelessly in love with Miriam. She seems different to me now, not an Indiana baby who came home with us, but *our* daughter who fits with us more and more each day.

"The Mir" or "Yum Yum" has changed, yes. She smiles, though almost invariably at her mobile and rarely at us (sigh). She is alert and interested in the environment when I take her on a house tour, which I do when I am trying to get a burp (the walking calms her). She stares at lights and loves patterns: her current favorite is the patterns made by the leaves on our ficus, particularly in the morning when there is sunlight on them. She is very normal, average, and that is comforting. No colic (though there is nightly fussiness), no digestive problems, regular poops (has our correspondence degenerated to that level already?!). Listening to the stories of women in the mothers' group and their problems with breastfeeding, colic, spitting up (she doesn't), etc., I can't help thinking how lucky we are. NO, not lucky: we have gotten what we have deserved for a very long time.

You are *not* the only woman in America without a baby. Next week a woman named Katherine is coming over. We connected through the adoption network. She is a freelance documentary maker who came to terms with her own infertility by doing a film for the local PBS station on private adoption. It was highly regarded, but I didn't see it because I had heard that it shows an actual baby being taken back by the birthmother. And you know, Lynne, that there are many others (still two couples from my adoption group who continue looking), but, of course, knowing and feeling are not the same.

I am SO pleased that you are working with a Golden Cradle agency. It is much safer and faster than international adoption. We had our home visit by *our* social worker the other day—I was not exactly fearful that we would not be approved, so spent most of the visit talking about your situation. She had done many international adoptions and echoed your concerns. She votes for the agency, if you've got the money. I hear it is hard to get accepted by one of those agencies, they are so in demand. What is the sense that you get?

Ms. M. has awakened. Did I write she is now eleven pounds and is almost three inches longer than when she was born? Yes, I do take her out . . . and glow like crazy when people, older women mostly, stop and coo at her and ask about her. I feel so normal I could scream as I walk down the block, "HEY, EVERYBODY, I AM A MOTHER!!"

Yes, she is cute; Rich thinks that she is beautiful. I am ambivalent, uneasy. Still not totally bonded. But she is good. She is, in fact, a *real* angel.

Love,
Barbara

NOVEMBER 20, 1986

Barbara,

Did I ever tell you that when I receive your letters, I never open them until I've performed a little ritual. First, I make a pot of tea, then I banish everyone from the room, and finally I settle myself into the left-hand side of the living room loveseat. I savor every word, sometimes cry, often laugh, and always read the letter one more time. Point being—no amount of envy will ever replace my *need* to keep in touch with you. Having said that, I do realize your life has changed and that time will simply not permit the luxury of lots of letter writing, so *do not* feel obliged to respond to everything I write.

Friendships are often so cyclical—most of the people in my life met a need or shared a common problem at one time or another, and yet in most cases I don't even remember the issues anymore. I guess those are real friends—the ones that are still around—and certainly you already fall into that category.

Regarding the "divine Miss M," I agree completely with Rich—she is beautiful! Such large, expressive eyes, and her little body seems perfectly proportioned. Have you any clue to what her coloring will be yet?

"Continuing to bond," you wrote, and I must confess to some amazement. I have always anticipated an *instantaneous* bonding, which I suppose is just my romantic notion of it all. It really does help, so much, to get glimpses of the next step via your experiences.

Regarding our progress—still not much news. LSS application and home study signed, sealed, and winging its way to the Philippines. Golden Cradle application being sent next week. In the interim, following up a lead from my brother about a brand-new agency in Albuquerque. My hopes, however, are pinned on the Golden Cradle. *God, how I hope!* You're right—money does provide more options, but it never made me fertile, nor does it now provide any guarantee.

There are already several inches of snow on the ground, which makes everything so difficult. Time now to put on my boots, to get to my car, to scrape off my windows, to inch through town, to pick up Annie. Poor Ken has business in Florida. Quite suddenly Ann has been expressing a lot of concern over the adoption plans. What a wonderful Thanksgiving you're going to have this year!

Love,
Lynne

P.S. I am P.S.-ing from a restaurant. I am to meet one of our district managers at 8:30 (it's now 8:15). No matter how hard I try, I can never arrive anywhere less than fifteen minutes early! As you reminded me, I was in a similar spot writing to you when Miriam was born. Can that really have been less than two months ago???

After I wrote to you last night, I got a call from Gwen, a woman from our six-couple LSS adoption group. One month after completing their application they have a baby. She is white, her husband black, and of course I know mixed-race babies are easier to find, but still . . . They were totally unprepared for the call and stopped on the way home from the agency (with the baby) to buy a crib. I wonder if I should start accumulating some things. It seems practical, and yet the thought of a fully furnished empty nursery fills me with dread. Kind of like not telling anyone when you're interviewing for a job you really want—for fear that you'll jinx it. Crazy, hmm? Damn, 8:30 and still no manager. Who are these people who are so casual about appointments? No doubt the same ones who fumble for change at toll booths, take forever to write a deposit slip at the bank, and get pregnant when they miss one pill! Crabby? Yes, I guess I am.

Later,
L.

NOVEMBER 27, 1986

Dear Barbara,

Seven-thirty A.M., day after Thanksgiving—very quiet here. Ken has left for his office (I'm off today), and Annie is still asleep upstairs. Wisconsin looks pretty today. Right behind our house are acres of farmland, and just about this time the cows come out after milking—a very interesting sight for a displaced city girl. The first time I saw them, I didn't have my glasses on (I am very nearsighted), and I screamed for Ken to identify the huge moving objects. "Bears," he replied nonchalantly.

We had a nice day yesterday. We boycotted dinner with the in-laws and asked no one to our house. Right before we ate, each of us went around the table and said what we were thankful for—and you might be interested to know that Miriam made everyone's list. I don't think I ever told you that I just knew Miriam would be a girl, and though I would gladly take either sex, I am, I admit, partial to girls. Despite a few typical problems, my mother and I have always had a good relationship. Mainly, I remember her coming in and talking to me right before I'd go to sleep. Sometimes weighty subjects, other times simply what I would wear to school the next day. I've kind of started it unconsciously with Annie, and she reminds me of "talking time" if I ever forget.

On Wednesday I mailed the Golden Cradle application, and naturally I've been torturing myself ever since. What if the price has gone up since I inquired? What if they've run out of babies? What if it gets lost in the mail? What if they've suddenly gotten a long waiting list? What if they go out of business just as my name comes up?

No one does "what if's" better than I do . . . Naturally, I will follow up with a phone call next week. I finally pried a copy of our home-study report out of LSS without having them drop me from their program. (They don't like to release these documents to the parents.) I had not seen it before. What a ridiculous document— poorly written, sugary sweet, and in no way a reflection of who we are; still, I am told this is typical.

Like the rest of the world, I am Christmas shopping today, so will close for now.

Love,
Lynne

DECEMBER 1, 1986—ALREADY!

Dear Lynne,

I was moved to tears by your last letter. It made me realize that my letters are as treasured by you as yours are by me. I too have a ritual when yours arrive. It is made easier by the fact that, when I worked *outside* the home, I always came home first (ahead of Rich) and so didn't have to worry about being interrupted when I read your letter. I would go through all the other mail, saving your letter for last and then, tea mug at the ready (yes, really) would read it s-l-o-w-l-y, sometimes titillating myself by stopping to mull things over before going on to the next paragraph. I am so pleased we have found each other, over and above our shared pain, for we certainly are worthy of each other's friendship.

We returned Saturday from three days in L.A., introducing Miriam to all of her grandparents. It was both better and worse than I expected. Rich's dad seems to be worsening. You must repeat everything at least three times to be understood. He seems quite withdrawn. . . . He got some pleasure out of his first grandchild (baby variety), but not a lot. He couldn't hold her comfortably, which was a disappointment to him, and she was very fussy—more than we had ever seen before (probably because of all the excitement) making it hard to be around her. . . .

Interruption, as Miriam began making "I'm hungry" sounds and then got fussy, so I took her shopping (car ride is a fabulous tranquilizer). There I was in a store, trying to decide what colors your kitchen has—never mind why—when this woman walks up and says, "Cute baby. You did good." I was about to explain that Miriam is adopted, when it occurred to me that I *did* do good, damn good in fact.

So I return home and there is your day-after-Thanksgiving letter with a picture of your kitchen! I guessed right and remember thinking to myself that I bet your house is in neutrals—beige and white and cream were my guesses. Your living room proved me right. It looks like a spacious and lovely home.

Your letter made me wonder if I should start this letter all over again. You spoke of everyone's mentioning Miriam as something they were thankful for. I hope you realize that we are thankful for Miriam, more thankful than there are words for. We call her Miracle Miriam and Magnet Miriam (because no matter where we are heading in the house, we both seem to end up where she is, staring down at her—irresistible). Though I am not at all enthusiastic about going through it all the second time, I would do it again to end up with such a treasure.

The next day, the day you wrote me, we went out to my parents' house in Santa Monica. I had not seen them in years. . . . I had forgotten how much they would have aged in the meantime. My mom looked a lot older but was basically the same. My dad was another story. His memory has gotten very poor. He asked several times how old she was, and when he finally asked if the baby was a girl or a boy, it just did me in. I just hope he can remember that at last I got what I wanted.

You asked about bonding. I have brought the subject up in my mothers' group, to get some corroboration of my own feelings. A couple, including the other adoptive mother, said bonding was instant; the rest said it took a while. So, clearly, being an adoptive mother is secondary in the bonding process, though I suspect it's less loaded if you are a biological mother. I remember my good friend Kathy going on and on in the hospital with her daughter Anna, then eleven hours old, about "Who *is* this person? Where did she come from?" Also, I think bonding was and is slower for me because of already having lost a baby. It felt very risky for a long time to love Miriam. We don't feel that way any more . . . especially since our lawyer told us that the state rejected Lily's and Robert's signatures as being given too soon after the birth and had them re-sign—which they did, with no problem. Incidentally, Lily is doing lots better and seems to be on the road to emotional recovery.

I am more than pleased that you are pushing for the Golden Cradle route. Have you already been accepted by the agency? I have my fingers and toes crossed that your baby will come soon. (I can't *wait* to share new-mother lore with you!)

Only took me two and a half days to get this written. Not bad. I think, however, the time between my letters will be stretching: Miriam is awake a lot more now and seems to be demanding attention. Or maybe I just can't keep away from her when she's awake.

Don't let the holidays get you down. Your dream is getting closer; *hold to it.*

My love. I salute you with a cup of tea.

Barbara

Dear Barbara,

Seventeen days and counting since I mailed our application to the Golden Cradle. Assuming we meet their initial criteria (whatever the hell those are), we will be billed for our first payment—writing a check never looked so good! This part of the process usually takes about thirty days, or so I was told when I called on days five, ten, fifteen, and this morning. Naturally, I am tearing my hair out while Ken has adopted (no pun intended) an infuriating "there's nothing more we can do now" attitude. Oh, how I want this to work!!!! Before Christmas would be perfect—keep those fingers and toes crossed!

I'm glad you finally took Miriam to meet her grandparents, though disappointed that it wasn't more satisfying for you. I must say that as of late, my family has really rallied around me. Yesterday flowers arrived with a card that read "hang tough—love, Dad." I cried buckets because they have finally acknowledged my pain instead of the old "things could be worse" routine. I guess this is one of the positive by-products of the adoption process that is always being touted in the *Resolve* newsletter. Grateful? Certainly—but I would have gladly skipped these "benefits" for a baby. . . .

Speaking of the *Resolve* newsletter, I can barely read it anymore. Every letter published seems to have a "happily ever after" ending that lately I have found hard to take. Surely there must be people who never got pregnant *or* adopted a baby—what happens to them? How do they feel? This month I contemplated responding to the infertile stepmother who wrote in. I sincerely empathize with her, but I have no energy for now. The only letter I ever wrote was to you, and I really cannot imagine being fortunate enough to find another such relationship.

Maybe next letter I'll have good news re: Golden Cradle—'til then.

Love,
Lynne

Barbara,

Just time for a very short note—but must tell you some significant news. Yesterday Ken and I drove to Chicago and, unannounced, planted ourselves in the waiting room of the Golden Cradle agency. We requested a meeting with the director and said (pleasantly) we were prepared to wait all day if necessary. Undaunted by a receptionist *and* secretary, we were finally ushered in at 11:00 A.M.

Bottom line: We were *one* of several *hundred* applications received so far this month. Christmas and babies—there appears to be a correlation. "How many will be accepted?" I asked. About ten. "Who determines acceptance?" She does. "How?" By evaluating the application and writing "OK" on it. "Would you like a pen?" Ken asked, and she laughed and said that won't be necessary. And then she wrote "*OK!*" I'm thrilled, trying to be calm, not counting my chickens and all that shit, but still—thrilled! Another home study. More meetings, but it feels good. More later.

Love,
L.

P.S. Watch for a package.

Barbara,

Opened your gift on Christmas morning and promptly treated myself to an entire pot of the peppermint tea. Delicious—and smells so good too! Thank you.

The holidays were not nearly as bad as I'd anticipated. Ken and I managed to spend a lot of time together *alone,* which was a welcome change from the usual family madness. At one point we threw all caution to the wind and drank a bottle of wine to "our last Christmas as just two." Premature perhaps, but it sure felt good.

Tomorrow I have an appointment with Lutheran Social Services. We have asked them to send a copy of the home-study report they completed to the Golden Cradle agency. But LSS won't let us participate in their program if we're involved with another organization as well. They want us to officially withdraw from their foreign program *before* they release our home study to the agency in Chicago. I have tried to explain that the Chicago agency is not a *certainty* at this point, but they have remained adamant on their position. The law requires them to give me a copy of the report (after all, we paid $2,500 for it!) but the Chicago agency will consider the report official only if it comes directly from LSS. Interesting "Catch 22," don't you think? No doubt designed just to make me crazy . . .

My letters to you are so often filled with details of the baby questions that I think I've neglected to mention another significant happening in my life. I have resigned from my job—effective January 9. I won't bore you with all of the many reasons except to say that from the onset I've been walking a tightrope between labor and management. My heart has been with the former, my paycheck coming from the latter. Naturally, from a financial perspective my timing could not be worse, but I feel *so* relieved and confident that something else will come up. I have had a few preliminary interviews already, though certainly nothing that could be considered a sure thing at this point. Anyway—think of me on the twelfth, my first day of liberation . . .

Have a happy New Year, friend!

Love,
Lynne

JANUARY 3, 1987

Dear Lynne,

Wow! I mean *WOW!!!* I am touched and flattered by your generous Chanukah gifts; I was speechless when I opened the box and eight gifts fell out. I'd felt very Jewish and put upon (by Xmas) this year, anxious that Miriam know her mother is Jewish. Your gifts added to the celebratory air I encouraged around the candle lighting—and opened a discussion with Rich about making future holiday rituals include both Jewish and Christian traditions. So you can consider *that* the ninth gift.

My favorites are the socks—so lovely to look at, toasty warm, and they stay up! (and match my teal slacks). And the Miss Manners book: *hilarious* and right on. Did you read the section on adoption?

I gave the coin-shaped chocolates you sent (they're called *gelt,* by the way) to Miriam along with a great developmental toy (more about those when your darling arrives) for Chanukah. I ate the *gelt* in her behalf.

You made the special holiday warmer. No surprise; you're a special friend. Thank you!

More to share, but no energy: I'm laid up with a stomach bug, but briefly—yes, I did know you were quitting. I am also ecstatic about your ballsy trip to Chicago and resulting "success," I hope. What are the "ifs" about it?

Finally, want you to know of a further result of the *Resolve* 1985 newsletter letter I wrote that introduced us. I've been asked to write an essay on infertility for an upcoming book on the subject. I'll try to write *several,* but the one I'll give most energy to already has a title: "Dear Barbara, . . . Dear Lynne."

Love,
B.

JANUARY 12, 1987

Barbara,

What a wonderful picture of you—you're gorgeous and so is the kid in the hat! I was amazed at Miriam's growth (so much, so fast) and taken by her expressive eyes. The picture is simply perfect.

My initial ecstasy over our trip to the Golden Cradle has now given way to an "I'll believe it when I see it" kind of feeling. Not that anything has changed since I wrote, but nothing has happened either. LSS has forwarded our home study and all other relevant data, and I assume those are being reviewed. Tomorrow I will make a follow-up call. Though we have made it past the first hurdle, we still are not officially *in*. Despite their hefty fee, they made it quite clear there is no shortage of applicants. Once approved and "on the list," I can wait in peace (well, I think I can), but until then I feel anxious, unsettled, scared. . . .

As scheduled, I left my job last Friday with a significant amount of fanfare. Most meaningful, however, were flowers sent to me from the union business manager! I take great satisfaction in knowing we had a good relationship. I spent my first day of unemployment cooking—a hobby of sorts that (she said modestly) I do very well. Still no word on my consulting job, but may know more by the end of the week. WAITING WAITING WAITING. You'd think with *all* of my experience I'd be better at it by now. More later—hope you're feeling better.

Love,
Lynne

JANUARY 15, 1987

Dear Lynne,

NO NO, you can't do this to me! You mean to tell me you didn't have the foresight to steal some legal pads from your office before you left? I have this nicely organized LYNNE file, filled with your letters on yellow paper. What am I supposed to do with these bits of notepaper and notecards you are sending? GEVALT, such a problem!

Congratulations on your unemployed status. I hope you are using the time to make yourself feel good. Having a lot of unstructured time is a challenge—or so I found during summer vacations. What do you plan to do with it? about it? You mention a consulting job. You hadn't told me about that. What? Where? Do you want it? Will the hours be what you want? I am also tickled by the flowers from the union. And intrigued: it must have been quite a careful balancing act you performed. Was that stressful?

I appreciate your compliments about the photo. I also wanted you to see my dad's paintings (he's an artist), not to mention Miriam and how she has grown. Isn't it amazing? We can hardly believe how *fast* it is all happening. (People in my mothers' group think I am weird when I wonder aloud if there is a drug to slow down the rate of physical development. They don't realize I am kidding. But after waiting so long, I just want it to go slowly, so I can savor every moment.)

So you're a cook, eh? I too love to cook—used to, anyhow. But living here in the heart of California Cuisine Hipsville, I have slowly stopped taking food seriously . . . at least not as seriously as a lot of people we know do. The crowner was the night Reagan was elected in 1980, when we sat around the table with three other couples and discussed the best restaurants in Berkeley. THEY did, that is; I was in the living room getting drunk, crying and screaming at the TV as the returns came in . . . all those wonderful senators defeated. I remember going back into our (former) friends' kitchen and berating them all for selling the revolution down the river for food. Now it seems funny, but boy, was I possessed!

This letter is really rambling. I didn't mean to get worked up over that event again. What I *meant* to say was that I am interested—genuinely—in what sorts of things you like to cook. Do lots of it now; I assure you, you won't have time after the baby comes. I have a great salad dressing recipe I could send you and a mushroom pâté that is a whiz in a blender or Cuisinart and never ceases to impress guests. Let me know.

I am having a hard time writing for the book of essays on infertility. I got halfway through the one about our correspondence and just froze up. Maybe it is because I don't have my letters to you, and I may need them in order to finish the article . . . and I am scared to ask for them because I don't think I could bear to reopen all those wounds. Yes, that's it. If I can't figure out a way to write it without my letters to you, I may just choose another topic.

You'll have to update me on the procedures at the Chicago agency. What else do they have to do before you are in for sure? I can hardly *stand* the suspense, so I can imagine how nutso you are. Is this long wait routine or what?

Miriam is over three months old now. This next four months or so are known as the euphoric phase (it ends when they start getting frustrated trying to crawl), and boy, is she in it. She is curious about everything, smiles at everyone, and is into exploring the sounds she can make. So we are awakened, between 5:00 and 5:30 each morning, by screeches that sound like she is being killed, but actually she is just having fun with her vocal cords. It is a riot. She can take an object we put in front of her face if she slowly moves both her hands toward it and then, of course, it goes right in her mouth. She also likes to put her hands around her bottle when she sees it and bring it to her mouth . . . except eye–hand coordination is not well developed yet, so the bottle's nipple usually ends up against her forehead or up her nose. Hilarious. Hold on, friend, you will have all this soon. In the meantime, there is nothing wrong with enjoying the fact that you can sleep in the mornings. I think of you often at 5:00 A.M.

So now you have time, and I am always in a rush to get things done before Miriam wakes up. Well, I look forward to lots of letters and will do my best to respond. Do keep my filing system in mind, however (kidding).

One more, very wise word:

> *Just to be is a blessing*
> *Just to live is holy.*
> —A. Herschel

My love,
Barbara

Dear Barbara,

The tea I made to accompany your just-arrived letter has barely cooled, and already I'm writing back. Time . . . yes, I have lots of it. Due to this newly discovered resource, expect longer letters and perhaps even answers to the questions you ask. On that note—"Was my job stressful?" You bet it was!

Today marks the second week of my unemployment, and yes, it is a challenge. I read, write, cook, and still find there are far too many hours in the day. The consulting position I mentioned is still far from finalized—I hope to hear something by the end of the month. Should it happen, I would work on a contract basis with area businesses to provide personnel training to first-line supervisors and managers. If this doesn't work out, I will simply have to find something else—I'm beginning to feel like Mrs. Ken, and I hate it! One little "keep busy" project I've initiated is organizing the hundreds of photos we have in hundreds of shoeboxes. So you, my friend, are now the lucky recipient of three treasures. Slices of my life, if you will. The first of me at age three, with five-member doll family, is sent as proof that I was raised to be a mother. The second is of me, Annie, and my mother, taken while Ken and I were dating, and the third—my wedding (with sister)—pretty gutsy, wearing virginal white at thirty, don't you think? Add them to your "Lynne" file.

Now—Chicago agency update: As requested, all paperwork has been sent. At our meeting in December we were told the next step was personal interviews with them in Chicago. Fine. But suddenly everything has come to a standstill. To date the director has not returned five of my calls and two of Ken's. Ken (ever rational) says she is a busy woman—I say bullshit! Something is wrong—but what??

I will continue to try to reach her this week; if I am still unable to by Friday, I will send a certified letter. Why is it always so hard? Interestingly, I don't cry anymore—the hysterics have been replaced with a dull ache. No more feisty anger, just a quiet kind of sad. Do you really think that someday I will be writing to you about the "euphoric phase"? It seems so hard to believe . . .

Well, back to my stove, where consolation is found in slicing and dicing.

> Love,
> Lynne

P.S. Legal pads! I knew there must be some reason why my usually organized life was feeling so chaotic. Rest easy, I will get some tomorrow.

P.S.S. One hour after completing my letter to you, my father called. An attorney he knows has a birthmother in Albuquerque!!!! No other details available. The lawyer plans to meet with the woman tonight and call me in the morning. I am trying to remain calm and failing. Too nervous to write, so I'll go out and attempt to run it off. I wish you were here. I am out of control.

Details soon—I promise.

JANUARY 25, 1987

Dear Barbara,

I'm having difficulty concentrating well enough to put words on paper but must share all of last week's drama with you.

An Albuquerque attorney (who knows my family) has found a birthmother. Actually, she and the birthfather found him—at the suggestion of a high school guidance counselor. They are both eighteen, Caucasian, and (at this point) certain that adoption is the route they want to pursue. The attorney called my father, my father called me, and since then the phone has not stopped ringing. After considerable agonizing, Ken and I have decided to go for it. The agency in Chicago still has not returned our calls, and this situation is as close as we have come to anything real to date. Once our decision was made, the attorney took over. He Federal-Expressed contracts to us yesterday which state that placement will be made with us in exchange for support (until delivery), medical expenses, legal fees, etc. Both birthparents have signed. We realize the contracts are not enforceable and all of the risk is ours—but surely they must at least represent a psychological step of sorts. Tomorrow Ken will wire our first check to the birthmother—$800 per month. The legal process is cumbersome in Wisconsin and will require two attorneys: one in New Mexico and one in Wisconsin—estimated total: $10,000! The baby is due May 20—the birthmother wants no contact before or after, and insists on an out-of-state adoption. Foster care placement would be made in Wisconsin. I am numb, dealing with all of the details—but scared out of my mind. When the contracts arrived yesterday, Ken was thrilled, but I burst into tears from fear!!! Can I cope if she changes her mind? I really don't know.

This letter is a mess—a jumble of facts and feelings that I hope you can make sense of. I will write to you every step of the way and hope that somehow I will be able to find some of the strength you have always had.

Love,
L.

JANUARY 30, 1987

Dear Lynne,

OHMYGOD. Your letter just arrived, and though Miriam is due to awaken any moment, I have to *start* this answer at least. It is a year ago precisely that Nancy's baby was born—yes, I am feeling very emotional and depressed—and now it seems to be your turn . . . *I am so afraid I will say the wrong thing,* I am so afraid for you. I am so excited that this may be it. I'm shaking.

My guess: They don't want contact and seem uninterested because they need to distance themselves from any pain—a really common response. Most people who disapprove of OPEN adoption think it will hurt all concerned if there is contact between the birthparents and the adoptive parents. I feel they are wrong; but while contact is often beneficial for the adoptive parents, the birthparents, especially birth-mothers, are another story.

Miriam. To be continued soon.

Evening: Rich is putting Miriam to bed, I've done the bottles and the dishes, and at last, time to put some thought to your situation.

What do I say? After having gone through it—twice—I still don't know what to say to encourage you. I still feel—I know I have written this before, probably back in our mutual trying-to-get-pregnant days—it is best to be prepared for the worst. And since you are so far from the birthparents, and I imagine will not meet them, you can distance yourself *somewhat* emotionally. Would you consider continuing with the Chicago agency, risking the loss of bucks? Feeling that you have an ace in the hole might help you survive the endless and awful waiting. And, anyhow, money doesn't hold a candle to the feeling of frustrated despair when you are left empty-handed.

The dreadful truth is that I have come to the conclusion that nothing birthparents claim about what they will do—this goes pri-marily for the birthmother—can be taken too much to heart until *after* they have seen the baby. I hate like hell saying that to you, Lynne.

What do you or can you learn about them? (If she's a student, why $800 per month?) Is the family of the birthmother supportive of her decision? Plans for after the birth? Going back to work? What? I will pass along all of Ellen Roseman's wisdom as you learn any facts.

Incidentally, this corroborates something Ellen told me when I told her your story. I haven't mentioned it before because you were in the midst of the LSS vs. Chicago agency business. She says there are plenty of ways for a resident of Wisconsin to get around the state laws about interstate adoption. I guess you have already learned that. So . . . if this one falls through, how about continuing on this route? Just a thought.

Rereading everything I have just written, it makes me realize I am being awfully negative. Wish to hell I didn't HAVE to be. But I wouldn't be your friend if I didn't tell you what I know and feel and what I am concerned about. (Yes, I am worried about their lack of interest, as you are. Maybe via the counselor you could suggest they read Suzanne Arms's *To Love and Let Go* and/or *Dear Birthmother* by Kathleen Silber and Phyllis Speedlin. Poor kids, they think they can just GIVE the baby away and forget it. Wrong.)

My letter is no more coherent than yours. I keep glancing at my calendar and thinking how *long* a time it is until May 20. If nothing else, you can write out all your anxiety and frustration and fears to me. I will be happy to respond and help in any way. I just can hardly bear the waiting myself; and I DO know what it feels like for you. (First, Pergonal empathy; now this. OY, maybe next will be empathy about the exhaustion and exhilaration of the 3:00 A.M. feedings. That'd be neat, for a change.)

Keep busy. Get a job. Think about an ace in the hole to keep you sane. And write. I am thinking and hoping and sending cool determination your way.

Hold on tight to each other.

My love,
Barbara

FEBRUARY 9, 1987

Barbara,

More than anything else this process is lonely! Maybe because of that I have changed my original plan of telling no one and have instead told everyone! Reactions vary, of course, but I've yet to find one that is satisfactory. If someone says "congratulations," I feel angry that they are stupid enough to be so premature; if they say "think positive," I feel I'm being patronized; and if they're cautious, I'm convinced that they believe it will *never* work. Needless to say, I'm not a whole lot of fun to be around.

Since my last letter I have not received much additional information. I have been told that to date all prenatal care has been received at a free clinic. On February 5 (at the clinic) she (birthmother) was assured that all was well and there was a strong fetal heartbeat. First appointment with a private ob/gyn is March 10. Birthmother is blonde (they say she looks just like me, but I think this must be some sort of learned-in-law-school line!), birthfather dark. She is a senior in high school and still attending classes; he graduated last year. I made a list of other questions, incorporated all yours, and called the lawyer this morning. He said he would get the answers and reiterated that she does not want to meet us. She did ask, however, if we would take the baby "no matter what." I said I was unwilling to say what handicapping conditions were and weren't acceptable and would reserve the right to decide at the time of birth. The lawyer said he would pass that along—but I got the distinct impression he did not feel this was a favorable response—and so we wait. I agree completely with your "ace in the hole" suggestion about the Chicago agency, but money is quickly becoming a problem. The first legal bill arrived last week; once it is paid and the Albuquerque scenario played out, our money is gone. To pay the balance of the Chicago agency fee, we would have to take out a loan. Yes, I know it's *only* money, but the prospect of having *nothing* to fall back on is frightening. But for now at least we will proceed. Despite all the craziness, I found I have made some personal progress. A friend called yesterday to announce her pregnancy (forty years old, first time), and I found I was not the slightest bit envious of her physical condition, only of how simple it seemed for her to get pregnant. I'm sure *you* understand.

On Saturday I have a third meeting with the consulting firm I told you about, and I'm very hopeful I will soon be employed. I really need to work. At home I remain obsessed from dawn to dusk, wearing only sweatsuits and rarely combing my hair. Add this to the permanent dark circles under my eyes, and well—even I can see that I'm becoming a mess.

I'm sure I'll write again before the week is out. Keep me in your thoughts.

Love,
L.

FEBRUARY 12, 1987

Dear Barbara,

Forgive me if this letter is redundant. My brain has been so addled as of late that I frequently forget what happened *when* and whom I've told *what*. So, with that disclaimer, I present the latest birthmother update. Her name is Christine. She does not smoke, drink, do drugs, or for that matter, use caffeine! For religious reasons, abortion was never an alternative. Her parents encouraged her from the start to place the baby for adoption, and once she came to that decision, she felt "100 percent better." Her parents have told her that once the baby has been born, she is welcome to come back to their home, and they will buy her a car and pay all college expenses. Christine plans to do that and is currently applying to several schools. She says she opted for adoption because she doesn't want to raise a baby on welfare and because she wants an opportunity for a normal life. She does, however, want to see the baby in the hospital because she is "curious." There are other questions I've asked that I don't yet have answers for—but Barbara, I am so encouraged. All communication is between the various lawyers, but I am consistently told she's committed to the placement and seems to have her act together.

I know, I know—everything could change following the birth, but for now, for today I am optimistic. I've decided to permit myself the luxury of believing it may finally be my turn. Ken, in case I haven't told you, refuses to be anything less than positive. He is discussing names, watching for crib sales, and sharing all of his child-rearing theories with me. I used to be afraid (secretly of course) that our adopted child might not be as special as his biological child, but I realize now, without a doubt, that that is not the case. We are both flying high—too high, I suspect—so feel free to include a reality fix in your next letter.

We continue to stall the Chicago agency. They've not called yet, but their bill still sits—unpaid—on my desk. In March we will have to do something with them.

Did I tell you we sold our house? Ken's company wants him to work from their Milwaukee office (an hour's commute), so we will move. I've started the house search but found nothing yet—though

I've been assured the market will pick up in March and April. Closing here is set for May 29 (yes, May—as usual, lousy timing), but we will manage.

I have found after five weeks that I miss my job—not the routine or massive amounts of work, but the opportunity to create change. On your advice I have looked for a job, but there is not much available around here. I'm still waiting to hear about the consulting job, but unlike you, I have no typing or clerical skills, so a temporary agency is not the answer. Almost every other temporary or part-time job is filled by students from the University of Wisconsin who are a huge and cheap labor force. So I spend a lot of time reading, writing, walking, and cooking—and, unfortunately, eating (would you believe—for two?). These days I'm into ethnic cooking—especially east Indian and Szechuan—anything with lots of garlic. . . .

Well, three teabags and seven pages later I suppose I should wrap this up. But before I do, I have to share a fantasy. The year is 2007. Miriam and "Elizabeth" (it's my fantasy, so it can be a girl—OK?) are sitting at a kitchen table reading hundreds of yellowed letters that all begin Dear Barbara, Dear Lynne . . . (sigh)

Much love,
Lynne

FEBRUARY 21, 1987

Dear Lynne,

Well, I thought I was past tears, but you really did me in with the vision of our daughters reading our letters. If I ever get past my writer's block, I will use that image to end my essay on our correspondence. (Is Elizabeth named after our mutual friend, the saint?)

The wall chart for measuring Miriam's height is adorable and so appreciated . . . particularly in light of the note you attached. When you wrote about finding yourself strolling absent-mindedly through the baby department, longingly fingering those tiny baby girl things, I was reminded of my days lost in fantasy as I strolled, heart aching, through the baby section of department stores. (Did I ever tell you about the time I almost lost it when Sears's loudspeaker announced, "Shoppers, there's a baby sale on the second floor"?) That you could pull yourself out of your blissed-out fantasy and still have heart to get something for Miriam is remarkable. But then, I have come to expect remarkable things from you.

Needless to add, I am excited about Christine. She sounds *as if* she is someone who knows her own mind. The lawyers sound *as if* they have a handle on Christine and have asked a lot of good questions. But I don't know for sure; that is the hard part. I think what I am trying to say is, be careful. God knows, I know how hard it is at a time like this to be cautious, but please try. There are always so many unknowns in open adoptions, and even more when you haven't met the birthmother. You know how concerned I am for your emotional well-being. Please keep me posted.

Aside from a last visit from the social worker (yes, to check for child abuse!), we are done with all the paperwork and visits for finalization of the adoption. It should occur in April. We will invite Miriam's godparents and my best friend here, Kathy, to come to our house for lunch. I am thinking that afterwards Rich, Miriam, and I will have a formal portrait taken to commemorate the day. She was given a totally gorgeous white knit dress (hasn't worn a dress yet; they look so silly on bald babies) with a satin collar, made in France, and I am hopeful she can wear it that day. I will let you know the exact date and will send photos. I am getting excited!

We are starting to childproof, as the M is on the verge of crawling: she scoots backwards . . . very common in babies who are just learning to go forward. She has discovered other babies and loves to go for their eyes. Got to watch her all the time. That's all right; I love to do it.

Lots of love,
Barbara

I finished this in one sitting—amazing!!

MARCH 5, 1987

Dear Barbara,

As you no doubt determined from my last letter (and despite your subsequent reply), my natural instinct for self-preservation has slipped. I'm afraid that the emotional investment in Christine is already so great that no amount of mental precautions will help if she changes her mind. So, I'm vulnerable, I know that—but are you really so sure that you crash harder from a genuine high than from a feigned neutral? Christine and birthfather begin sessions with a social worker this month. They will talk at length about the adoption decision, as well as provide a complete medical history. A report, summarizing the sessions, will be sent to me. I'm hoping this will provide additional insight—but who knows. As I recall, your first birthmother seemed the epitome of well-adjusted. So "it ain't over 'til it's over." . . . *Of course,* I will call you just as soon as the baby is placed in my arms— or upon my release from the local asylum.

Your newspaper picture and announcement of Miriam's adoption was great. The other one (at your parents' home) has been framed and sits on my desk, but my favorite remains the homecoming shot in the rocker.

I cannot believe Miriam has yet to wear a dress. How can you resist all of those sweet little outfits? (Damn—these days a smocked bodice alone reduces me to tears.) Bald babies are adorable, though I must admit to a bias. Family legend has it that I was a dead ringer for Eisenhower until age four.

Your adoption party sounds great—I envy your proximity to the end of the road (at last). Your letters, photos, and unsolicited advice are cherished.

Love,
Lynne

Barbara,

Lots of news.

Last week I spoke at length with Bev, the social worker who has been seeing our birthparents. She is a wonderful woman who is both sensitive and candid. It seems much of my original information was wrong (I don't know why), but I now feel fully informed. As I was told before, they are seventeen and eighteen years old. Birthmother is English-Irish, senior in high school, and raised Catholic. Her father is a career army officer and loathes her boyfriend. He is the one who said she must leave the house until after the birth of the baby, but her mother is in frequent contact. Believe it or not, *her* parents are both thirty-eight years old—*can you stand it?????* Birthfather is from Spain; came to New Mexico with family at age three. He's a high school graduate who recently joined the army. They had discussed marriage, but Christine decided against it. Per social worker: "She is quite mature for her age—good grades, anxious for college, and despite pregnancy has no desire to completely alienate herself from her family." Bev says she seems totally committed to adoption! Birthfather much less mature but, to date, willing to go along with what Christine wants. He is currently stationed in Texas but will be given a pass to sign all necessary papers upon birth of baby. Bev confirmed that Christine does not want to meet or speak to me, but she did want a letter. I wrote four pages yesterday describing us, our home, and our interests. She may or may not write me back, but she *will* write a letter for the baby.

Anyway, I feel good, I really do. Assuming there are no problems with the birthfather, I think we're home free. I know that makes you nervous—and it does me, too—but Barbara, it feels right and good, and for now I want to enjoy the anticipation. If it all falls apart, I'll live and continue—just as you did. Despite my general optimism, I continue to hold back a little and still have not (nor will) purchase all the wonderful baby-related things I want. *Don't worry about me—at least now.*

Also, since my last letter, I have gotten a temporary part-time job. I'm doing management training, on a contract basis, with a local nursing home. Once I've put in my paid hours, I've made it a daily practice to volunteer some time. During those hours I just visit with the residents, and this experience has truly made a difference in my life. Melodramatic perhaps, but it feels so good to give something to someone. Yesterday a ninety-seven-year-old woman told me, "I like you so much because you touch me when you talk to me." Who would think a hand on a shoulder could mean so much. I guess what I'm trying to say is—I feel pretty good about me!

Wrote this letter in record time, trying to beat the mail carrier. More soon.

Love,
L.

MARCH 15, 1987

Dear Lynne,

Rich has taken Miriam to L.A. to visit his dad on his dad's birthday. I have opted to stay here alone for one reason: I wanted and am enjoying tremendously a weekend all to myself . . . amazing to realize how much stress there is in just being constantly responsible for human life. Yes, I know: you have no sympathy for that. Someday you'll understand. Won't that be great?

So yesterday I slept late, went clothes shopping for the first time in six months, and went to a movie (*Little Shop of Horrors*—overrated). Today I will start cleaning out our mess of a basement, do some cooking, and go have a solitary hot tub before picking Rich and Miriam up at the airport. (In the back of my mind all the time, however, is a fear of plane crashes.)

A kind of routine has developed around here. Monday morning I babysit Kai, a boy six weeks older than Miriam. On Wednesday mornings Kai's mother reciprocates, and I run errands . . . and sometimes just sit in the living room and relax and think. Thursdays I meet with my original mothers' group (we alternate mornings and afternoons to accommodate the women who have gone back to part-time work), and Friday mornings is the community college mothers' group (the rainbow group, I call them: several welfare mothers, immigrants, and a few middle-class types like me. I enjoy the variety). Friday afternoons Kai's mother, who is also in the community college group, and I take a long walk in the park with our kids. So, I am busy: I didn't expect to be, and I like it. My proclivity for joining support groups has introduced me to a lot of interesting people.

Sometimes, though, I wish it were otherwise. There are issues in my future that I need to think about. Like, a part-time job: if not teaching, then what? I know I will want time away from Miriam (I know, it makes no sense to you), but doing what? The idea of a job search makes me nauseous. The other issue is kid number two. I guess there will be one, but going through the whole thing? YUCK. Not to mention my anxiety over whether I'm going to be too old to handle two toddlers. And . . . well, I'll stop there; you don't need to hear this right now. After you have your baby, maybe we can write about it.

Miriam has TWO TEETH!! We finally figured out why she was waking in the night and having a nonstop runny nose. Teeth. Amazing . . . and no more toothless grin. I am filled with nostalgia.

She is trying to crawl. She gets up on all fours and rocks back and forth; "revving her motor" we call it. She has a genuine laugh now. She is starting to get more hair; think it will be a light brown. She is becoming *very* active; I will have my hands full when she starts to crawl. Got to childproof this place one of these days . . . before it is too late.

I am thrilled that Christine and birthfather are going through counseling. Is that mandated by New Mexico? Great idea. If she is a good counselor and gets them to think about what it will feel like afterwards, then that is a real plus. Nevertheless, nevertheless, nevertheless, you remain in that terrible state; I guess there is nothing I can do for you except be here for you no matter what.

Touch of reality for you: If you put a dress on a baby girl, you put tights on underneath to keep the legs warm, yes? Then you have to take them off and put them on again six or seven times a day during diaper changes . . . and babies get squirmy awfully fast.

Have you thought about a boy? Name? Circumcision? (I thought a lot about that one—it is a toughy for a Jew, lemme tell ya.)

We don't know when the finalization will be, though most assuredly within the next six to eight weeks.

I have never written you about the agreement we made with Lily when we were in Indiana. We have been writing and sending pictures every two weeks. (I'll write her after this letter is done.) Starting when Miriam is six months old, we will write once a month. We will renegotiate at Miriam's first birthday, but I would guess that it would go down to three or four times a year. She writes about as often as we do. She is *planning* to come for a visit in July, but since she has been laid off for months and earns a very low salary, we are unsure if she could actually afford to make the trip (driving and with the girls, too). I want her to come. I think it is important for her—and all birthmothers, if they can—to visit the home to see for herself that she made the right decision, that everything is just fine, and that we are a family. It will put her at rest about what she did, and that matters to us, too.

What's the due date? How are you keeping busy these days? Keep busy!!!

My love,
Barbara

MARCH 16, 1987

Dear Lynne,

I haven't felt this shit-kickin' excited about someone else's state of mind since I don't know when. Your letter was full of such good news . . . and hope, that I just can't maintain my stance of "I'd better keep cool so I can help Lynne out if it is needed" anymore. It sounds excellent; let's get excited together.

I am excited mostly because you have never written sounding so upbeat, so positive before. This is the Lynne who hasn't been around much since this correspondence began (two years ago yesterday, by the way). Now I KNOW we are going to be mothers together . . . by hook or by crook. I just finished wrapping your gift, which has been at the back of Miriam's closet for over a year. I thought I would never get the chance to wrap it. Felt great. One day or the other it will be on its way to you and your baby. HOTSHIT!

And now I know you too are a survivor. I can sense your deep drive and determination and reservoir of strength which will carry you through whatever is to be. And I rejoice for all of that.

Bev sounds excellent, and that is solid GOLD in this business. I am also encouraged by what she passed on about Christine and the birthfather. All I want now is to know that Bev is discussing with Christine what it will feel like afterward, the grief, the emptiness. And encouraging her to plan for it and prepare herself and family and friends to be there for her.

Wonderful, wonderful, wonderful. Sorry our letters crossed in the hands of our postman, but glad Miriam slept long enough for me to get this off.

Keep the faith.

Barbara

MARCH 18, 1987

Barbara,

Christine changed her mind—marrying birthfather, found out March 17. Despite all your warnings, I wasn't prepared—it hurts. It hurts a lot. Ken's been great, and I'm at the airport now awaiting arrival of my mother, who is coming to hold my hand. I'm so sad, so disappointed. Can't write more now, but will send details.

Love,
L.

MARCH 20, 1987

Barbara,

By now I assume you have received my postcard regarding Christine's change of mind. It is, I realize, nothing compared to the pain you suffered the first time, but it hurts nonetheless. Damn—it hurts!

The change of events was caused, I am told, by the birthfather's mother. She visited Christine regularly and encouraged her to move in to her home and keep the baby. It is rather easy to understand (given the alienation from her own family) how this idea could have become appealing. During the week of March 8, Christine discussed the possibility with Bev (the social worker). Bev called our attorney, and he called Ken, saying "Things were becoming shaky." Ken told me nothing—hoping it wouldn't happen. Finally, on the morning of the 17th the attorney called Ken again, saying it was over, and Ken left work to tell me. I was shocked, amazed, devastated. I was also angry that Ken had not kept me informed, though I am convinced it was done with "good intentions." Because we had stupidly announced everything to everyone, we had to unannounce it too. The "sympathy" calls and trite reassurances were unbearable—but I guess the worst is now over. My wonderful mother flew in, made endless pots of tea, and just listened, a godsend.

As if all this wasn't lousy enough, the Chicago agency (the "ace in the hole") is now being investigated by the Illinois attorney general and rumored to be closing. So it is back to nothing once again. I have not (*will never*) give up, but I am tired and discouraged. Currently my plan is to move (4/25/87), find a house and a job, and simply start over. It appears as though we will have to put our things in storage and stay in a hotel for awhile, as my house hunting was significantly delayed during the recent happenings. Continue to use the same address; mail will be forwarded.

Our attorney has filed suits to recover our money from the birthfather and Christine's parents (because she is a minor), but we're not very optimistic. Two thousand seven hundred dollars had already been paid in attorney fees and that is gone forever, but perhaps we will get some of the monthly expenses back; I don't know.

Though I know you will take no consolation in being right, *you were:* I should have been more cautious. Next time (*and there will be a next time!*) I'll remember.

Much love,
Lynne

P.S. Minutes after finishing this letter your beautiful tulips arrived—my favorite—thank you so much! Someday, my friend, I am going to give you the biggest hug you have ever had—I promise.

L.

MARCH 27, 1989

Lynne,

A friend has taken Miriam. When I told her about you and why the mail made my mood catapult, she wisely offered me some alone time to grieve, rage, and try to find the right words. So, here I sit in the Everyday Café with a pot of Earl Grey and two chocolate cookies, one for you and one for me. I'm pretending the empty seat across from me has you in it (as I did one tearful day in a hot tub) . . .

It should be wine instead of tea. There are no sober words in me to ease your pain. Here I am on the other side of that grief, and in spite of my experience, I find no easy way to help.

So: *Grieve. Rage.* Throw things. Get drunk if you need to; I did. *Vegetate.* Do whatever you need to; give in to what you feel. You get it out of your system, and then, you get tired of it. You pick yourself up and then keep busy. I knew my jobs, my days, my shopping trips were just time fillers, distractions. But I got to prefer them to just vegetating. Do what you need to do; you'll get to that point, I promise.

Let Ken, your mom, and *you* (most of all) nurture and care for you.

And write me . . . when you want to and can.

Oh shit, I love you, I grieve for you. I never get used to life's unfairness; I'm so damn mad.

And I am thinking of you. I'll never give up till you're a mother.

Love,
B.

MARCH 29, 1987

Barbara,

By the time you receive this letter, I will be on my way to Albuquerque. There are a number of papers that need to be signed regarding our legal action against Christine, and I am meeting another birthmother. Given the recent disappointment, I have been hesitant to mention this second "opportunity" (even to you), but I find, as usual, I need your support.

Bev (our social worker) was so distressed about Christine and us that the very next referral she got, she turned our way. This woman is eighteen, has a thirteen-month-old baby, and is pregnant again. She has recently broken up with the birthfather, who is a thirty-five-year-old married policeman. I have spoken to her on the phone, and she has requested a meeting.

Ken is not enthusiastic and believes we need a chance to recover before jumping into this process once again, but I am compelled to follow up—particularly given the situation at the Chicago agency. Maybe I am crazy, but I simply have to go!

My phone conversation with the birthmother, Carrie, was rather tense, though we did share a laugh about our common anxiety over all of this. . . . I told her about our recent experience and plan to discuss it again, at length, when we meet. Should anything come of this, we could use the same attorneys—on both sides—and I assume, similar financial arrangements, though this woman lives with her mother and presumably would not have such big expenses. This time I have told no one and, I believe, am grounded in reality. Still, hope springs eternal and all that shit, and I just have to go. I am scared out of my mind, but strong and determined. My trip to Albuquerque is scheduled for the week of April 6—think of me and send me strength. When I return, we will move. Still haven't found a house, but we're continuing to look. We will rent an apartment, I guess, and that will have to be home for awhile.

Annie came up last night for the weekend, and we (finally) told her about Christine's change of mind. She was stoic through the entire discussion (as was I), and then she went to her room and cried. When she came out, she came and sat by me on the couch and said, "Would it help if *I* called you Mom?" She is a sweet kid, and I know she feels my pain. Well, friend, I best close. It is important to me that you know what is going on—I really need you now.

My love,
Lynne

APRIL 10, 1987
ALBUQUERQUE, NEW MEXICO

B — met with Carrie last night. She is bright, attractive, and surprisingly mature. Says she has chosen us as the adoptive parents. She seems confident about the decision and is already in counseling with Bev. Many more details to be worked out, but we will proceed. Ken still very cautious, me intact—but so scared. Leaving for home tomorrow—long letter to you then. I feel your concern.

Much love,
Lynne

APRIL 13, 1987

Barbara,

Crazy time again . . .

Moving men have infiltrated and are packing and crating all around me. When they come for my desk, I'll have to stop writing this letter, so bear with me as I attempt to cover a lot of ground quickly.

My trip to Albuquerque was very positive, for a number of reasons. First, because I met Carrie. Regardless of what may happen, the actual experience of meeting a birthmother is not one I will soon forget. Carrie seems mature for eighteen and (though I hate to say it) confident that adoption is the best solution to her problem. The birthfather is thirty-five, married with three other children. Carrie has had a relationship with him since she was fifteen (!) and already has one other child (twelve months old) that is also his. For some time now, he has told her he will leave his wife, marry her, and live happily ever after, but after two years of excuses she says she no longer believes him. She says having a baby is not what she expected, and she cannot deal with a second one as a single parent. I told her my story—up to and including our last disappointment, and in an hour and a half I really think we developed some significant rapport. The bottom line is, she has chosen us; the lawyers are drawing up an agreement, and I am holding my breath. We exchanged names and phone numbers and will stay in touch until the birth (late June). We are wary, cautious, and yet—as ever—hopeful. While in New Mexico, I met Bev (the social worker), who has been so good to us. I trust her and know she is doing all she can on our behalf. I also fired our first attorney, who it seems totally screwed us over financially (details on that in some other letter) and retained the most experienced, well-known adoption attorney in Albuquerque—a woman, but of course! I have stopped trying to predict what will happen. I will stay in close touch with Carrie, but I will also proceed with my life.

Tonight we check into an apartment—a tiny, one-bedroom furnished arrangement that will be home until June 1. We bought a house in a suburb of Milwaukee but cannot get in until then. My resumes are being printed, and I start my job hunt on Monday the 20th. I'm trying—oh how I'm trying—to be prepared for the worst.

The movers are coming my way so I must close, but not before I tell you that your strength traveled over state lines and kept me sane while in Albuquerque. Do keep in touch—I need you now.

Love,
Lynne

APRIL 17, 1987

Dear Lynne,

I like what I read in your last letter. There's Lynne. She's back, folks. You are ready to risk, but you are not on some high-flying cloud. You are taking charge of events (as much as one can in this crazy business), and even more I read that you openly are presenting yourself and your feelings—to both that blankety-blank lawyer and to a real-live, flesh-and-blood birthmother. Congratulations. You've come a long way, kid.

I don't think there's anything else you can do. You have found yourself some good professionals. I am so pleased you will be working with the social workers you trust so much, and that you have found a well-regarded adoption attorney. In looking back, I think that being in the right place *emotionally* and having competent people whom you trust are 50 percent of the battle. The rest is chemistry among you, Ken, and Carrie . . . and fate.

And you are taking care of yourself "as if" it mightn't work out. The job hunt—I'll bet it's fun to put on all those pretty clothes and makeup, but I'd also be willing to bet that it is just something you are doing while waiting for the baby. Hey, whatever gets you through the day (and night).

Carrie's due date is in late June. That seems like a long time to me. It must seem an eternity to you! But you are lucky. You have so much to keep you busy: moving twice (ouch!) and the job search. The end of June will sneak up on you. In the meantime, all you have to remember to do is keep in contact with Carrie . . . and write me! I'll be on pins and needles till I hear from you again.

Love,
Barbara

APRIL 21, 1987

Dear Barbara,

My first piece of mail at our temporary address—a letter from you, as I knew it would be. We moved in last Tuesday, and all I am able to say about this place is that it is shelter. A ticky-tacky tiny arrangement with loud neighbors and several cars in the process of engine overhaul in the lot below. The rental agent says we are lucky to have gotten the unit with the sculpted shag carpeting (in shades of rust and green, no less). Ah, yes—lucky indeed!

But—six weeks and we're out! We bought a 1920 Georgian colonial that needs a lot of work, but with significant charm potential. Hardwood floors, leaded glass windows, and French doors. I'll send a photo.

As planned, I have initiated my job search—resumes sent, appointments made, and five suits dry-cleaned and hanging in my closet. Still, as you wrote, I harbor my secret fantasy. Bev called yesterday, and so far so good—via Bev: Carrie has requested a meeting with Ken, so he will fly out in late May. Bev will also have a meeting with the birthfather.

I think I mentioned in my last letter that we were had, in some respects, by our previous attorney. His fees (all prepaid) were outrageous compared to others in the area, and the support we gave Christine was very high (again, compared to other typical, local arrangements). We have requested a rather hefty refund from him, and if he doesn't come clean, we've been advised to go to the ethics committee of the New Mexico State Bar Association. To date his only response has been to imply that I am a crazy, obsessed woman who is looking for a scapegoat for a crashed adoption. This *infuriates* me and has fueled my determination to get him and a baby (though, of course, not in that order). Can there be anyone lower than those who exploit another's desperation?!

You're right—my attitude is good and my courage at an all-time high. Now if I can just maintain until June. A few miles from this apartment there's a beautiful park. During the day it is empty, and I've begun taking solitary hikes on a regular basis. Observing nature and all its wonders convinces me that everything *is* possible.

Much love,
Lynne

P.S. Don't forget to send details and photos of Miriam's adoption day—April, right?

APRIL 29, 1987
Miriam is seven months old today

Dear Lynne,

I have just twenty-five minutes to write this, before I have to get ready for my friend to bring Miriam back home. We take turns babysitting on Wednesday mornings. The few hours when Miriam is with her often turn out to be the only time I can do things like write letters, houseclean, pay bills, etc., so I have been running around like a chicken with its head cut off.

Things here are coming to a conclusion after years and years of dreaming and hoping. I feel a bit numb. On May 11 at 9:00 A.M. local time we go to the City Hall of San Francisco and appear in the chambers of Judge Arata. Our lawyer assures us that it will all be over in ninety seconds. A mere formality, but I assure you I can do a lot of crying in ninety seconds. We are getting all dressed up (yes, M will be wearing her first dress) and going with my good friend Kathy and the Tobeys, M's godfamily. Then we will return here, where Ellen Roseman will join us for a blowout lunch I have planned: oysters and champagne, poached salmon and asparagus, with a magnum of Rich's fine chardonnay which he made in 1983—the year this whole journey began—a platter of strawberries, and a chocolate cake from the best bakery in town, with more champagne and toasts. I plan to get pleasantly looped and do a lot of crying and laughing.

This is an amazing age. We no longer feel that we are caring for this lumpy little thing. We now feel there are three people, three personalities in the house. M is alert, curious, and filled with giggles. Wonderful! She is now about eighteen pounds and almost twenty-eight inches long. Crawls like gangbusters and has just learned to pull herself up, using anything she can. I have to remember not to sit in a chair near her, or stand near her unless I plan to be there for a long time, because she will instantly grab my pant leg and pull herself to a standing position. Sometimes she lets out a squeal of delight when she is finally upright. Hasn't learned to get down gracefully yet, but does a hilarious plop on her rear when necessary, and then crawls away. She has also started getting up at 2:00 A.M. and demanding food and then demanding to play. We are struggling sleepily with this new reality.

Love,
Barbara

MAY 6, 1987

Barbara,

I'm hoping this letter arrives on May 11, to be read after your guests go home and you've finished your champagne and oysters. Because just in case you've not heard it enough today—congratulations!!!

You did it, kid—you really and truly did it! It gives me goose bumps just to write that and a vicarious sense of exhilaration. You beat the doctors, the lawyers, the doomsayers, and the statistics—you made your dream happen, and I'm so very proud (and weepy, I might add) to have been a part of it! Your victory renews my admiration for womankind. We are so strong and smart and tenacious. So forgive me, Rich and Ken, but *you* did it, Barbara, and soon I will do it too!

I feel much more in control these days. I am ready (and only too willing) to put aside all of the last few years of disappointments. You, I also note, have also done that. That is not to say that you don't remember—I know you do—but you're not angry anymore, though thank God you're still sarcastic.

I spoke to Carrie last night on the phone, and everything appears to be progressing well, but of course, I worry. She says she now tires easily and is so anxious for "it" to be over (*No shit!*). John, the birthfather, has met with Beverly, and that too was uneventful. He said he would have preferred abortion. I spoke to Bev and told her I was a bit concerned over Carrie's matter-of-fact attitude—she seems so detached and la-de-da about the whole thing. Bev says I'm never happy (so what else is new?). We're going to Albuquerque on May 28 so Ken can meet Carrie. He was to go alone, but I've decided I need to be there. Ken is cautious and skeptical, but willing.

I've still not landed a job here, but I've gotten a few temporary assignments to fill my days, the last of which should end June 1, which coincides to the day with our house closing. Yes, yes, yes—the house is lovely!

Don't forget to send pictures from adoption day.

Love,
Lynne

Mother's Day card:

My love and admiration far outweigh my envy—even now . . . Enjoy your day—you've earned it!

Love,
Lynne

MAY 13, 1987

Dear Lynne,

You will be pleased to know that your imagined scenario for Monday worked out just as you'd hoped. The last guest stepped over the pile of mail that had come through the slot and left. I picked up the mail, poured myself one more glass of champagne, and opened your letter. How delightful and intuitive of you to have thought that far into my special day!

Like all great moments in life, it was uneventful and somewhat of an anticlimax . . . but very affirming, as your Mother's Day card suggested it should be. We were in the judge's chambers for ninety seconds, as Larry said would happen. But in those ninety seconds the judge did say M was a beauty, which was nice. M's godmother cried, my friend Kathy insisted on hugging everyone, and Larry handed M a gift and a beautifully written letter. We (Rich and I) each were sworn in and agreed to allow the other to adopt Miriam. Then we traipsed to the recorder's office to have the papers certified and filled out a request to the state of Indiana to send us a birth certificate with Miriam's *new* name on it.

Then we came back here—we had decorated the house with crepe-paper garlands and long yellow irises (my favorite)—and the Tobeys and Kathy and Ellen Roseman and we had a meal, replete with toasts . . . and a tearful one by me. I also raised my glass "to all the women out there who are on the road to this destination, especially my friend Lynne." Miriam got some lovely books as presents (I hadn't expected that). Everyone left by two; I read your letter and then just plain collapsed.

Five years. Five damn hard years. It all came crashing down on me, that it was over. I think this is what is called postadoption depression. I cried and cried and then slept for the rest of the afternoon. I have been a zombie since then. I've spent two days stretched out on the couch, watching Miriam and sleeping when she sleeps. I'm in a kind of shocked, dazed state. Though it is not *bad* per se, it just feels like a process I have to go through to get my balance back.

Tomorrow my mothers' group meets here, and we will have

champagne and cake all over again. They are all very excited for me and will want to hear the details. Part of me wonders when and if they will ever see me as just another mother. (That same part wonders when I will see *myself* that way!)

I am marking the days until you and Ken go to Albuquerque to meet Carrie. I am sure it will go well; no doubt Ken is a warm and charming man (to match his wife) and will do well with Carrie.

Now then, unsolicited advice, part two: I'm with you. I am uneasy about Carrie's "la-de-da" attitude. Does she know, has Bev talked with her, about what it will feel like afterwards? How she will mourn, grieve? How hard it will be? Is Carrie willing to hear this? She needs to be pushed to talk and think about IT—how does she want things to go in the hospital, who will be there, how will you and Ken first see the baby, hold it, receive it from her? What about future contact: How often does she want phone calls and photos and letters? Best to negotiate all the delicate stuff in advance. The best advice Ellen ever gave us was this: Don't pussyfoot around. Don't be afraid to ask for things from your birthmother. If she can't tolerate that, better it should fall apart *before* than *after*. (I'll vouch for that.)

Bring her a copy of *To Love and Let Go* by Suzanne Arms, a book about women who've relinquished and their emotional states, as well as relationships with adoptive parents. If you can't find a book called *Dear Birthmother,* let me know. We gave it to both our birthmothers. It is written by two women who worked for Lutheran Social Services in Texas and is a collection of actual letters from/to birthmothers from/to adoptive couples. They aren't literature by any means, but the book successfully conveys the feelings around open or semi-open adoptions. It will give her a lot to think about . . . like, does she want to write the baby a letter explaining *why*? (I think that is a really good thing for the child's mental health.) Very hard to find, but Ellen has a stack of copies, and she will get me one for you, if needed.

I don't suppose you could arrange a flight through S.F. on your way home?

How goes it with the first attorney in Albuquerque? Any success yet in that situation?

It's worth repeating that the next six weeks will go fast with all you are doing, and I am glad for that. I am thinking of you and sending strong-woman vibes, but it seems like you got plenty of those going for yourself. ALL RIGHT!!

Love,
Barbara

P.S. We all had too much champagne to remember to take lots of pictures. But whatever we have, I'll send.

MAY 19, 1987

Barbara,

Once again your "unsolicited" advice was well timed. I *have* been pussyfooting around with Carrie regarding the tough issues. I think I had some crazy idea that if I didn't bring those up, maybe she wouldn't think about them, and then maybe she wouldn't change her mind. I realize that's nonsense now, and I do have a plan. I have drawn up an agenda of subjects that will require decisions. I will call her tonight to introduce them and insist that we come to some agreements at our meeting next week. Hopefully, the lead time will prevent the rather vague "I don't know" that I typically get in response to my questions.

You asked about lawyer number one, and I'm happy to report we received a refund from him last week. We also received a snotty little letter about his deep concern over our "misplaced grief"—spare me!!!

As you continue to note, I *am* stronger this time. However, not so strong that I won't crash hard if . . . so am I really in control or simply more adept at appearing to be? I'm not sure.

One wonderful diversion is our new home. I am immersed in obtaining bids for redecoration and choosing paint, paper, and furniture. Enclosed is a photo (fuzzy because Annie took it, but clear enough so you'll get the idea).

I've also had two job interviews—though no offers yet, which frankly suits me fine, for now.

I'm glad your adoption luncheon went so well. I could feel the celebration from here. So your story is over—yes, hard to believe. I know this is a *very* premature question, but do you really still intend to do it again sometime?

As much as I would love to come home from Albuquerque via San Francisco, I'm afraid it won't work. We leave Thursday night (5/28); Friday the 29th we meet with our lawyer, then Bev, and then we'll have dinner with Carrie *and* her mother. The 30th we return home. I'm nervous, excited, and eager. Ken is nervous. Can't wait to write you all the details. 'Til then—

Love,
Lynne

JUNE 1, 1987

Barbara,

Just time for a very short note while awaiting the moving truck. Our trip to Albuquerque went (dare I say it?) exceedingly well! Our Friday evening dinner lasted four hours—we laughed, cried, and addressed every agenda item. So far, at least, there has not been a hitch. Just before we concluded the meeting, Carrie said, "Look, Lynne, your baby is moving," and I felt him (or her) and cried. Whoever is in there already feels like mine. Ken was wonderful—he was charming, confident, and cool throughout the entire meal and then promptly threw up once we arrived back at the hotel. So much for macho.

As soon as I am a bit more settled, I'll write you more of the details. The due date remains the same (July 4), so one way or another it will be over soon.

Love,
Lynne

JUNE 8, 1987

Dear Lynne,

This should catch you right in the middle of the organized chaos of the move. I hope it is going well, that you grow happier and happier getting to know your new home (the third since I've known you!). Rich and I were both blown away by the photo you sent. That is a fabulous home.

I'll write quickly, because I have to pick up Miriam in a few minutes. This is the one day each week when I am home alone, and I had hoped to get tons done, including a long letter to you; but fierce cramps intervened, and I have spent most of the day on my back on the heating pad. YUCK.

I sent lots of support your way during the short time you were in Albuquerque. It sounds like a rapport was set up and there is the beginning of a long-term trusting relationship. I hope . . . Ya never can tell; keep telling yourself that. Nothing counts until she has seen the baby.

I feel good about your situation. Whether it works out or not, you are clearly in a good place and will survive. Nevertheless: keep busy and prepare for a disappointment.

You are surprised that we are planning to go through it all again. From the place where you sit now, it should make at least a *little* sense: we survived, and we know we can survive again. Plus, we have a greatly reduced load of "baby lust" now that Miriam is here. She would be our comfort if something fell through. My concern—aside from where we will get the money—is what effect it would have on Miriam if the birthmother changes her mind. But all this is a long way in the future—over a year at minimum.

My mind is drifting, thanks to too much codeine. Maybe I will stop and try again tomorrow. Or just mail this off and ask your forgiveness for such a short note.

Love,
B.

JUNE 16, 1987

Dear Lynne,

First I got angry at the postman on Saturday. I spent half the day standing at the front window waiting for him to come . . . I repeatedly told Rich that there was a card from Albuquerque for me in the mail, and I couldn't wait to get it. There was *no* mail delivery that day! The card arrived on Monday, and I really glared at him when he came. *Then* there was no mail delivery yesterday again—I mean no one got any . . . and I knew that was when a letter from you should arrive. The postman is lucky I wasn't home when he delivered today.

I did in fact send powerful support signals your way all last week, thought about you a lot . . . though, to tell you the truth, not with a great deal of anxiety. From your letter detailing what had transpired with Carrie, it is clear to me that you hit the ground running and have gotten in touch with your internal reservoirs of determination . . . and courage (to mix a couple of metaphors). I am a lot less worried about you. You are now at that place I was a few weeks after Nancy took the baby back: I was astounded by how my determination was fed by my outrage. I've thought about it a lot since then. Decided it actually brought out the best, the strongest in me. I don't think I . . . or you . . . are unusual, really. We are very normal people with fairly healthy self-regard, and we know when we've been had, boy. And we get up and fight back . . . Hooray for us! You're gonna make it, kid.

As to Carrie: Well, you never know . . . but I am encouraged by the fact she has another child, so she must be very reality-based about parenthood. No image in her head of a pink-dressed angel who never poops or cries at 3:00 A.M. That, and the fact that she is seeing wonderful Bev, encourages me a lot. I am a little edgy that she has continued to see the boyfriend for so long . . . hope she isn't doing the adoption bit in the hope of getting him back.

And I am encouraged by *your* attitude, though I know the pain you feel and the secret fantasy about all this that you aren't sharing with anyone, and your stark terror . . . I remember, and I feel it for you. Have had a stomachache ever since your letter arrived . . . a very familiar kind of stomachache.

I encourage your attitude of carrying on with your life, job hunt and all. You will be busy in the weeks to come with that and moving, and I am glad for that.

Most of all I am encouraged by you. You are going to get what you want, by God, that's for sure. If it's not this one, then the next, or the next. You have suffered almost the worst of it, I think. Someday, SOON, before this year is over, you won't have to hold tight any more . . . except to your dream which will be your reality at last. Yes.

My love,
Barbara

Ju ne 1987
Resolve *Newsletter*
Feedback

Her letters are treasured . . .

Two years ago, on a whim, I responded to a letter to the Editor, and gained (much to my surprise) a friend for life. I've never met my friend or even spoken to her, but her letters have become my source of strength, and treasured reminders of our shared path to parenthood.

Through sheer determination and commitment, my friend now has her baby. Her example consistently gives me the courage to carry on. I can think of no better way to pay tribute or give thanks than to return to the place where we met. Bless you, Barbara Shulgold!

Lynne Sipiora

JUNE 15, 1987

Barbara,

I loved the adoption pictures. You really are a beautiful family! Amazed (as usual) at Miriam's growth—it goes so fast, too fast . . .

Thanks for the compliments re: the house. I am still convinced it *will be* fantastic, but right now it is anything but. Since our arrival I've been living with an army of contractors—everything needs something—the kitchen is completely nonfunctional and the general environment, chaotic. The major projects, however, should be completed by July 1. We feel confident that someday we'll be able to realize a big profit, but for now I just want to settle in and live.

The countdown, of course, continues here, and interestingly, I'm calm—very calm. I guess I finally realize that there is simply nothing more I can do. Bev is meeting with Carrie today to go over the hospital procedures; our check for the hospital bill has been sent to our attorney's trust fund. Annie is with us so that she can go along when the time comes, and my brother is sitting by his phone. I can't remember if I told you about Ron's (my brother) role. Assuming all goes well, the baby will be released at twenty-four hours after birth to Ron (who lives in Albuquerque). At our attorney's suggestion, we will not come to the hospital or anywhere near the baby until the papers have been signed after seventy-two hours. I understand this precaution, but I hate it!

I've still not purchased anything and will not until we finally know. Keep your positive thoughts coming my way—I'm close, really close.

Love,
Lynne

JUNE 17, 1987

Dear Barbara,

Nine A.M. at the Covered Bridge Stables; Ann is taking her first horse-back-riding lesson, and I'm playing suburban mom—schleping and waiting—oh yes, and waving from time to time . . .

I think it was just yesterday or the day before that I wrote to you that I was "calm, cool, and collected." Welllll, not anymore. I am a wreck—the baby has dropped, and the birth is now expected within ten days!! I spoke to Carrie's mom last night and was told she is very worried about Carrie and how she will really deal with this. Though, of course, I've been worried about that too, her comment drove it home again. It is still a long way from over. I have been keeping busy—still much to do at the house—but not so busy that my mind doesn't wander. Just after I hung up the phone with Carrie's mother, a man called and asked to speak to Ken. He was a sixteen-year-old birthmom's father and heard about us from my East Coast aunt. It was a rather vague conversation, but it does give me hope that if this doesn't work, there will be others.

But damn—I want this one!!

My bag is packed, with your phone number safely tucked inside. Think of me.

Love,
L.

JUNE 21, 1987

Dear Barbara,

We have just finished our final coat of paint. The kitchen is up and running, there are geraniums in the outside planters and even the beginning of an herb garden—so I'm ready, damn it, but Carrie is not!

For about an hour last week we thought it was time. Carrie called Ken's office and said the contractions had begun. I packed my bag, steeled my nerves and, of course, the contractions stopped. Since then—nothing. We are so close, and yet it remains far from over. When I called tonight (I've been calling—at Carrie's request—every other day), I spoke to Mary (C's mom); she said Carrie was spending the night with John (the birthfather) and that he's been "hanging around a lot lately." Naturally this concerns me. Though he is not available for marriage, he clearly has a helluva lot of influence.

Despite my best intentions, over the last week I've given in to positive anticipation. Birth announcements are addressed and ready, and nursery furniture is on order (though there is an option to cancel until July 15). My parents have postponed their vacation, and Ken's mother calls daily for a delivery update. How can I cope if Carrie changes her mind? Will I have the inner resources to attempt all this again? I feel a significant anxiety attack coming on—hold on. Well, I really have no other news at all; every day is spent the same—waiting, and there are only so many ways you can describe that in a letter. Happy Father's Day to Rich.

Love,
Lynne

JULY 2, 1987

Barbara,

I swear this *really* *is* the last letter you'll receive from me before showtime.

As of yesterday, Carrie was well and showing no signs of delivery. Her doctor, however, insists it will not be long—his guess: five days. As the time draws closer, Carrie appears to be "bonding" (?) with me! I've not decided if this is good or bad. Anyway, the result of this happening is that she wants me in the delivery room and will release the baby from the hospital only to me. This, of course, totally ruins our plan for having my brother get the baby and for us to attempt some measure of self-preservation. So, bottom line—I'm going to Albuquerque tomorrow afternoon with Annie. Ken will join us as soon as her labor starts. We could be there three days or three weeks—who knows! I know this letter is disjointed, but I have so many last-minute details to attend to; still, I couldn't go without a letter to you.

The picture of you and Miriam on the night you came home is in my wallet. I look at it often.

Soon—dammit—soon!

Love,
Lynne

P.S. Ken has stopped throwing up and is now wringing his hands over the cost of college, which should coincide with his retirement. When worried, he cleans, and he is currently scouring the tub, which is just fine by me, as my reaction to stress is to take to my bed. I'll call.

Healing

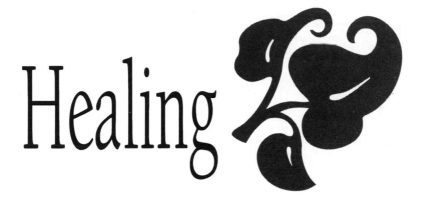

Lynne:

On July 6 Elizabeth was born. As planned, I was in the delivery room with Carrie, and the doctor handed me this beautiful baby girl seconds after she was born. She was warm and she was real and she was mine. The hospital staff was wonderful—I bathed her with the help of Annie and my brother, who had sat in the hospital lobby all evening. We called Ken from the nursery and took turns screaming into the phone, "It's a girl, it's a girl!"

At 7:00 A.M. the following morning, Annie and I picked Ken up at the airport and drove directly to the hospital. Moments after Ken was introduced to his new daughter, the staff pediatrician called us to his office. He felt he had detected a heart problem and indicated that an immediate consultation with a cardiologist was necessary. Elizabeth was taken by ambulance, and we followed behind in the car. Ninety minutes later the cardiologist informed us that Elizabeth had a congenital heart defect that could not be corrected and would die. . . . We returned to the hospital, and I went to Carrie's room. After long discussions with Carrie and her family and the staff, it was decided that Carrie would stay in the hospital with the baby and we would all go home. There was nothing anyone could do. I said goodbye to Elizabeth in the nursery and marveled at the happiness she had brought us—even for so short a time. We arrived back in Milwaukee at 9:00 P.M. that night, and at 10:00 P.M. I called Barbara for the first time.

Barbara:

July 7, 1987, is warm in San Francisco. I know all my friends are outside enjoying the weather. So when the phone rings, it has to be Lynne. I run down the hallway in my stocking feet, almost spinning out of control as I fly into the bedroom.

"Yes? Hello?"
"Barbara, this is Lynne."
"Lynne, tell me."
"My baby died."

We had an unspoken agreement that we wouldn't talk to each other until we both had children. So the first phone call is far from the conversation *we had both anticipated: Lynne's voice is thick with tears and too much wine; I am barely able to mouth words of comfort. The call ends with tearful promises to write soon.*

HALF AN HOUR AFTER
OUR FIRST PHONE CALL

Dear Lynne,

No sleep tonight. I keep thinking about you there, alone and angry. I hate feeling so helpless, so useless. I wanted to say the right thing, to give you great comfort, but, as a wise and loving woman once wrote me:

There are simply no words. I have cried for you, my insides are torn apart, my heart is broken and the tears still won't stop. If I could, I would carry your grief for you—because you have had enough. You are constantly in my thoughts.

You don't have to write at all. But I will.

Barbara

JULY 8, 1987

Dear Lynne,

Today is harder for me than last night was. Is it harder for you? The light of day makes your tragedy seem more real, not just a nightmare. There is a piece of icy cold steel cutting through my intestines.

My craving for chocolate, usually reserved for the day before my period, is enormous. I spent much of the afternoon walking the streets of San Francisco, stopping at any store that might have chocolate bars. I even went to one twice, feeling like an addict.

For no accountable reason I burst into tears this morning. It just hit me like a whip. I played the St. Matthew Passion, last played the day our first baby was taken back, and had a good cry; but I don't feel much better, knowing how much, much worse you must feel . . . and wondering what I can do to help. Just write, I guess, as usual, and blather on, in the hopes it will at least make your grief a little less lonely.

I spoke to Ellen Roseman. She has given me the names of a couple of women in her adoption service who have had tragedies similar to yours. I am waiting for a call from one. I will feel her out, and if I think she is sensitive enough for you, I will ask her to drop you a line. I hope you don't consider this too audacious.

Just like when a favorite aunt died many years ago, the sky is clear and summer blue today. UNFAIR. I would have wished you the endless gray rainy days I got last February when Nancy took the baby back. I appreciated the fact that nature wept with me. You don't have nature's cooperation and sorrow, but you have mine.

You'll hear from me again soon. You'll get my love and concern whenever you need it; I think of you and send you courage all the time. Count on it.

Love,
Barbara

JULY 9, 1987

Barbara,

Since returning home, I've just kind of stumbled around in a haze. Lots and lots of phone calls from people who truly care. Ken has been concerned as I tell the story over and over again, but for some reason that has seemed to help. Elizabeth was mine for less than a day but that short time reaffirmed that this quest is worthy of all the pain. Yes, I will try again—though I'm not sure when. Our lawyer called yesterday to discuss yet another birthmother, and though I was tempted, I'm smart enough to know I cannot deal with it right now.

Ken has been wonderful, despite the fact that I totally pulled away from him for awhile. Something kind of snapped in my head when I watched him comforting Annie. For about ten hours I hated both of them. After all, they had each other, so the loss was mine alone, but I know now that isn't true. I remember Ken holding Elizabeth with tears streaming down his face, asking the doctor how we could make her well—and I remember Annie kissing her over and over again. She was such a sweet little baby. Perfectly formed little body, dark curly hair, and big feet. I don't know, Barbara, was she *my* first baby? Was Nancy's baby your first?

Tomorrow Ken will go back to work and Ann will go back to her mother and I will get on with my life. I know I have to get a job—for distraction and for money. Medicaid will pay Carrie's medical bills and the baby's, but there are still legal fees, air fare, etc. . . . She and her family were warm and caring and truly seemed concerned for me. There are so many feelings I need to share with you, but for now I am just too sad. I'll be okay, I guess. As always, I appreciate the fact that you are there for me.

Lynne

P.S. I wish I hadn't been so fuzzy with wine and tears on the night we finally spoke. Ken asked what we talked about, and I really couldn't remember—then—or now.

JULY 9, 1987

Dear Lynne,

I have just had a most extraordinary conversation with an extraordinary woman. I have rarely talked with someone so wise, so deep, so compassionate. I felt a little bit like a child sitting at the foot of a wisewoman and learning the secret of life—or rather, the secret of living your life.

Jane and her husband adopted a boy, Michael, at birth. He had a severe heart problem, and, to make a long story short, had a heart transplant but died at eighteen months. Since then they have almost adopted two children, one (I think) with a severely emotionally dysfunctional birthmother, and another with physical problems. Both adoptions fell through at the last moment. They have gone through intense grief therapy and have come out the stronger for it.

More than that, she is a sensitive person and speaks so articulately about losing babies that—well, what can I say—I was bowled over. I hope you don't object, but I have given her your address. She said that she will write you next week and would very much like to call and talk to you. I would urge you to reach out to her. She has a tremendous amount to offer. I don't have your new phone number, so I gave her your old one. I hope that is all right. Please trust me on this; she is a special person . . . my gut reaction is that she is the person you need to talk to when you are ready. She (and her husband) really want to talk to you . . . and Ken, if he wants.

She was also very concerned about Annie, as am I.

You continue to be in my thoughts. I can feel your pain today across the miles.

I liked her phrase "honor your grief." Do that.

I'll write again soon.

Love,
Barbara

JULY 13, 1987

Barbara,

Today, a week since—we are beginning to recover. There are still moments, of course, but by and large we are functioning and back to all the day-to-day routines. Sometimes the entire Albuquerque experience feels more like a dream (make that nightmare) than reality. Was I really there? Did I really hold that baby? Her little face is already starting to fade, which is perhaps nature's coping mechanism. Carrie's family held a funeral on Friday, and my wonderful brother, Ron, attended. He said Carrie was a mess—hugged him and said only, "Tell

Lynne I'm sorry." I am truly concerned about her and imagine she is experiencing a hell of a lot of guilt (i.e., "It wouldn't have happened if I hadn't decided to give her up"). Ron said the ob who delivered the baby was also there. Anyway, it's over. Ken has talked to Carrie since, but I've not been able to yet. As you might imagine, we have now received the sympathy vote from every social worker, doctor, lawyer, etc., everywhere. Already we are being told about other birth-mothers, other possibilities. Ken has stepped into the leadership role and I've stepped out. I do not know what the future holds, but I do know somehow–some way–someday, we will try again.

Same day—noonish.

Two letters arrived today from you. Wonderful, sensitive letters that convey (once again) how much you care and understand. I will, of course, speak to your friend. Shit, I'll talk to anyone who might ease the ache that seems to have become a permanent part of me. Strange to me how my grief doesn't seem to show. I've been through a life-altering experience, but at the grocery store and gas station, I'm just the same old person. Once again my mother has offered to come out (they live in Florida), but, though tempting, I've declined the offer. Her presence would simply provide another excuse for wallowing about even longer. And—already I'm tired of suffering. Since my Tuesday evening call to you until yesterday, I was either in bed or wandering around the house crying—undressed, unbathed—awful! And frankly I scared myself. Everyone has a point, I believe, where they've gone so far they can't get out—and I was close. So close that the shock of recognition frightened me into fighting it. So I guess, friend, this is strength and (want it or not) I seem to have it. I will survive.

Annie appears to be OK. Ken has spent hours talking with her. She has returned to her mother's home, but before she left we shared a special time. I have four antique rings from my maternal grand-mother—one is mine, one is for the child I will have someday, one I gave to Carrie just after Elizabeth was born, and the fourth I gave to Annie when we returned home. I told her it represented a legacy of strong women and that her strength and courage helped me—because, even more than Ken, she was there for it all. Then we held each other and laughed about how we raced to the hospital in a car I didn't know how to drive, over desert roads we'd never seen. And we chuckled over how the hospital personnel must have thought we were the strangest team on the maternity floor—me gowned and in the delivery room—and my eleven-year-old stepdaughter and her uncle pacing the waiting room. Then we cried as we recalled meeting with the cardiologist and were told Elizabeth would never come home. The hospital gave Annie (unknown to me) the baby's footprints, and she asked if she could keep them. . . . I think it's okay for her to remember the baby in any way she chooses—don't you?

Funny, I didn't think I would want to write again, but I do and it does help.

Love,
Lynne

JULY 15, 1987

Dear Lynne,

You write that you don't remember much of our phone conversation, but I do: you said you were through with searching for babies. I had to remind myself over and over during the next few days that you were in the first stages of grief and should not be taken at your word. But I did worry. It sounds like you are both beginning to do grief work, and I am glad . . . and even gladder that you are not throwing in the towel, as tempting as that might be at the moment.

When my best friend Kathy walked through the door the night the baby was taken, she threw her arms around me and sobbed, "Oh God, now you know what it's like, what it feels like to have a real, warm, responsive baby in your arms, now you know how *wonderful* it is." I have to say the same to you. Now you know: that makes losing the baby even harder; but, I hope, it should also make you more determined to find your baby. It is an awful way to reach that determination, I know. But the alternatives? Unthinkable (I hope).

You asked if I felt like Miriam is my second baby. I wrote on the card sent to you and our other friends that our first baby had been taken back. However, you might notice that now I only refer to her as Nancy's baby (you should have heard me yell the night Rich made the mistake of referring to her as Miriam). No, she is/was not our child. She has another name now, and Miriam—the only one there is or will be—is asleep here in her crib.

But your case is different. So damn different. I don't know what to say: If it helps to say that she was your first child, then say so. Just as long as it doesn't make the grieving process harder. I just do not know what to tell you. If you choose to consider her that way, remember that you can still name the next one, should it be a girl, Elizabeth.

During our conversation you also said over and over that you had to know *why* it happened. "I am too intelligent not to understand," you said. My personal opinion is hopelessly modern and agnostic-sounding. I don't believe that things happen to us for a reason; they just happen. The trick is getting over them, past them (the bad ones, that is).

A friend told us it was *bashert* (a Hebrew word meaning "fated") that the first baby would be taken back, because how else could we have found the baby who was "looking for" us, Miriam? A nice romantic notion, but I don't believe it. I think all life is wondrous and worth our love. There are so many babies out there for you to love. I won't give up until you have found at least one.

Another book worth reading is Harold Kushner's *When Bad Things Happen to Good People*.

You say that Ken is concerned about your telling the story over and over. Everything I read suggests that that is one of the best ways to work through grief. I did it myself. I remember the first time I went to my mothers' group, with four-week-old Miriam in my arms, and cried as I told the story of the first baby . . . and a quiet voice inside of me said, "Thank God, I don't *need* to do this anymore." I think resolution of grief is accomplished in part by sharing (there is in fact an organization called Resolution through Sharing, for the parents of children who died).

You can tell me the story . . . and about your rage and your emptiness as many times as you need to. I will be your sounding board as you were once mine.

You might want to consider having a ritual of your own to "let go" of the baby. Perhaps a solitary hill and the releasing of a balloon. Whatever . . . I just wonder if some sort of ceremony mightn't help. It is up to you.

I worry and wonder and talk of you and to you every day. Write when the energy is there.

Love,
Barbara

JULY 23, 1987

Dear Lynne,

I did not mean to let a week plus elapse between my letters, but responsibilities have overtaken me. I had wanted to write very often, so that you wouldn't feel that—after all the initial consolation calls— your grief was forgotten. I have felt very guilty about that, so I am especially relieved at the contents of your last letter. You are beginning to function normally again . . . I am impressed at the speed of your recovery. (You're not pushing yourself, are you? That would inevitably backfire.)

What extraordinary behavior the men in your life are showing! Has your brother always been so wonderfully compassionate and generous? Would you consider renting him out to me as an ex officio brother? Men like that should be declared a national treasure. And your SWEET husband: the experience is deepening him, sharpening his sensitivity, I'll bet—though he has always sounded like a man who has learned from life's dark side and grown. I know it is no consolation to you, but you are fortunate not to be totally alone in this tragedy.

Well, you really got me with those rings. It sounds to me like your grandmother gave you a far greater gift than just the rings . . . and you are passing on that gift with great, open love. I pray that Carrie learns a bit from you . . . and from the tragedy she is enduring.

And Annie—how can she help but survive it with two adults so sensitively attuned to her welfare?

So, as you can see, your last letter produced a prolonged sigh of relief here from both of us (I read parts to Rich; he now asks daily if there is a letter from you).

A small note of warning: The grief may come back now and again (less frequently as time heals) and wash over you like a relentless ocean wave. All you can do is stand firm and wait for it to pass.

Like yesterday: Larry, the lawyer, called. It seems the social worker called him and informed him that he had never filed the form cancelling the petition to adopt Nancy's baby. He wanted me to know that he would do it right away, and that it would only take him about forty-five minutes (read, $75). I just freaked: found myself throwing every toy I could get my hands on down the long hallway. I was amazed how much of my anger, my sense of *outrage* returned. "That bitch, she haunts my life still," I screamed. I called him back and told him I didn't want to spend my money on such an insulting and hurtful bit of bureaucratic nonsense. He, mostly concerned with maintaining good relations with the social worker, said he would do it at no charge. Small victory, but I spent the rest of the day wanting to go smash Nancy's head in, and finally broke down in tears. After all this time.

But it's the next day, and it is all gone.

Thinking of you. Really, I am . . . a lot more than my letter writing would suggest.

Love,
Barbara

JULY 26, 1987

Dear Barbara,

I'm feeling better, and it's mainly because of your birthday. I was wandering around downtown today kind of aimlessly looking in store windows when I happened upon a dusty little antique shop. It looked deserted, which was appealing, so I went inside. To make a very long story short, it was there that I stumbled upon the antique purse which is your gift, and Henry Lowenstein, the owner and proprietor. Somewhere in the midst of examining his wares I found myself telling this little old man my whole story up to and including Albuquerque. He listened intently, urged me to sit down when I got a little teary, and even served me tea in a delicate little antique cup and saucer. Telling Henry was cleansing in some way, and I left feeling better than I have in days, thanks to the "kindness of strangers." So Happy Birthday, Barbara, from me—and Henry.

Love,
Lynne

JULY 29, 1987

Dear Lynne,

As it happens, Rich's present to me for my birthday was a pair of tickets to this Saturday night's San Francisco Symphony production of the Mozart Requiem, a favorite of mine. I can hardly wait to strut around in the magnificent new Davies Symphony Hall with my new out-a-sight purse. It's stunning. You have a fine eye.

And a wonderful heart. How very like you to remember someone else at such a dreadfully hard time in your life. And to have made a connection, too, with Henry—who sounds like a mensch of the first order for lending such a sympathetic ear.

How are you? Are you being good to and gentle with yourself? It's our motto, remember! Are you forgiving yourself bad moods, backsliding . . . and getting it all out of your system?

And how is Ken? I really do want to know. He must feel so . . . useless. My best to him and from Rich, too.

I'll be thinking of you at the symphony Saturday night as I sparkle with my new sparkly evening bag. Thanks again.

Barbara

JULY 31, 1987

Barbara,

Carrie called me Monday evening, and we talked for almost an hour. She has grown from this experience and seems to be making some positive plans for the future. The conversation was rather unemotional—though I did ask her at the end if she had ever contemplated changing her mind. Perhaps during delivery or right after birth? She said, "Never," and I believe that.

Tuesday, I relapsed. Spent the entire day in bed crying. Tortured myself by reading the journal I'd kept, looking at the birth announcements I'd made, and walking in and out of the empty nursery. Wednesday was much the same, Thursday better, and today OK. I knew I wasn't finished with my grief, but I didn't expect it to return with such force.

In the meantime, we have received another call about the birthmother in New Jersey (it seems *no one* gets pregnant in Wisconsin), via the connection from my aunt. I refuse to get involved, but Ken has had two conversations with birthmom's father. I've asked him for no details, and he has said only, "It would be a real long shot."

Sooner or later I know I have to gather my internal resources together and attempt the whole process again, but I'm just not ready yet.

Tomorrow we leave for Florida. My father sent three round-trip airline tickets, and we've decided to take advantage of the change in scenery. A week's worth of ocean and beach couldn't hurt.

Yes, my brother always has been sensitive and wonderful. His sense of family love and loyalty go very deep, and I am ashamed that I've never fully appreciated it in the past. Nowadays, however, I keep getting a mental picture of our departure from Albuquerque: a hot and busy airport, crowds everywhere, and this big man (6'3", 200 pounds) with tears streaming down his face saying over and over, "I just want you to be happy, Lynne." Gives me goose bumps even now, and reminds me (again and again) how much I love him.

Not one member of my family has let me down over the last month. Another lesson learned (as always, the hard way).

Love,
Lynne

AUGUST 11, 1987

Dear Lynne,

Sometimes I wish there were a computer that I could attach to my brain that would write down automatically all the letters I write to you in my head. I just wrote you a great one, as I lay on the couch with my eyes closed . . . have no idea if I can remember it all . . .

. . . but it began with an apology for what in retrospect was a slightly breezy thank-you note for my beaded purse, filled with encouragement for your doing so well lately. Thinking about it, I remembered how I had my good and bad times for months after our tragedy. You have a right to the bad times. I hope you will share them with me, as well as the good ones. Don't let me or any other smartass take away your need to grieve at your own pace.

I think about you a lot, a lot. I think how lonely you must feel . . . even I have deserted you in a way. I talk to you in my head and say just the right things. They evaporate into thin air when I am confronted with the damn typewriter.

Of course, I cried when I read your letter about your conversation with Carrie. I guess it would have helped to know she might have kept the baby. On the other hand, now you have another valid reason to grieve, if you need another one. I am glad you allowed yourself to collapse after that. I think you are on the road up and out of the worst now. I hope so.

When THE BABY THAT STAYS comes, she or he will erase most of the pain and almost all of the memory of Carrie's baby. Nancy's baby does *not* exist, just as surely as Carrie's doesn't. She simply is not the person she would have been with us.

I am outrageously impatient to share motherhood with you. We will, of course; I just want it now . . . and painlessly, too. You are right to take your time, to nurture yourself. And you are absolutely right to refuse to take part in following leads. Your husband . . . what can I say. His actions speak volumes about his character and his devotion to you. Give him a hug from me, please.

This is not the letter I wrote on the couch. For me it is ending in tears and an empty feeling, a loneliness. I hope to hell it did more for you. I love you.

Off to the Sierras camping until the 22nd.

Love,
Barbara

AUGUST 17, 1987

Barbara,

Our week in Florida went fairly well. My parents were concerned, supportive, and (like so many people) optimistic about the future. Despite the obvious good intentions, the latter grates on me. Optimism is only for the innocent.

One night, however, my mother told me that my brother had talked to her in detail about Elizabeth's funeral. I had never wanted any details. Anyway, it seems Carrie changed Elizabeth's name—which was certainly her right to do, but I felt devastated by this piece of information. I'm trying to understand my feelings, and I think my latest grief is my inability to even know how to grieve. How do you mourn the loss of something you never had? Is it the baby I'm crying for or the return of my own frustrations and longing? If I'm honest, I think the latter. After the cardiologist examined the baby, we were all ushered into her office. I was the last to enter (holding the baby), and she (the doctor) was behind me. I remember vividly that she squeezed my arm hard and whispered to me, "It's very bad." And in those few seconds Elizabeth was already gone. Naming her had at least validated the experience in some way. Now a baby is dead—a tragedy—but though I ache, I have no real claim to it.

My gloomy intro aside, I have taken a major, positive step since my last letter. I got a job! I saw an ad, got my professional shit together, and forced myself to apply. Three interviews and a psychological assessment (my luck, I'm still sane) later, they made an offer. So, effective August 24, I will be the personnel director for a local health organization.

Please save your congratulations—for though I'm pleased to have a paycheck and a place to go, I'm also very depressed by it. It seems symbolic, somehow, of the end of the line, a return to the childless, professional couple we once were and may always be . . .

This week before I begin work is a quiet one. Ken is in Denver on business; Annie is back in Chicago for the start of school. I thought I had a lot to do, but I can't remember what it was anymore. I continue to avoid all baby leads, so Ken fields calls and letters. Yes, yes, yes, he is a wonderful man! Maybe the reason all this happened (yes, I still want a reason) was to show me just how devoted he truly is to *our* cause. Okay, so maybe that's a result, not a reason, but I'll gladly settle. As always, your letters help. Please don't feel you shouldn't mention Miriam. I love the details of your motherhood and the milestones of your daughter. First step, first word—I'm hungry for it all.

Love,
Lynne

SEPTEMBER 6, 1987

Dear Lynne,

If I'm lucky, this letter will reach you on your birthday, at least partly taking the place of the present which will arrive late. I know you probably feel you don't have a lot to celebrate right now, but I feel you do: you have survived so far . . . take it from me, that says a lot.

You have a lot to struggle with, but I hope you will take some time out to congratulate yourself.

And you've got a job! I can't believe you went through all the rigors (interviews, etc.) and grabbed the job to boot. You must really be something! (Actually, I know you are.)

Just reread your letter: "Please save your congratulations." Well, I blew that. BUT you do deserve to be congratulated, for not throwing in the towel on life completely, and for at least getting yourself out of the sitting-around-the-house-in-your-bathrobe-blues. It will keep you busy . . . that is probably the best thing of all. I *would not* have survived the nine months "between babies" if it had not been for my low-stress job.

You write that you resent all those well-meaning souls (family?) who say, "Now, now, dear, don't fret. You'll have a baby in no time, you'll see." Yup, I remember that. That is so hard to hear. But, Lynne, you *will* have your baby . . . you HAVE to. Besides, I have no intention of allowing you to go childless. AND I have already bought the present!

What I would never say, and will never promise, is that it will be easy. There are no guarantees that the worst might not happen again . . . and again, though it is unlikely. It is a hellish business, and I am here for you to sound off on until it is finally over. Actually, let me restate that: The worst might happen, but it will not affect you in the same way . . . first, because you have survived such a tragedy already, and second, because you will guard your feelings closely.

You sensitively give me permission to talk about Miriam. I was hoping you hadn't noticed, but I have been unable to write about her since your tragedy. Are you *sure* you want to hear? I feel very uneasy about this, since I remember all too well my own jealousy and anger after the baby was taken back whenever I would hear about anyone else's baby. Well, okay. I tried to give her a bang trim last week and she moved: now she looks like a punk toddler. It is awful! Rich keeps saying she will outgrow it, and of course he is right . . . but I keep trying to get her to wear hats. No way; she hates them.

Last Friday night Rich and I were sitting in our living room easy chairs, about four feet apart. Miriam was standing and kind of leaning one elbow on Rich's thigh when she suddenly gave me a big smile, reached out her hands, and toddled over to me. Did you hear Rich's and my screams of joy? We were beside ourselves with excitement.

She got up and did it again, this time eighteen steps . . . but who's counting? We ordered pizza and had champagne to celebrate. We let her stay up an extra hour so she could continue to "practice." It was fabulous . . . and what everyone had told us seems to be true: this (walking) is the one stage babies seem to recognize as exciting, too. She smiled and laughed the whole time.

Lily—and daughters and new boyfriend—is talking of coming out for Xmas. I am nervous, ambivalent . . . though I feel it is good for all concerned (except me). We'll see if she does in fact make it this time.

I am sorry it took so long to answer your last letter, but Miriam is now taking later and shorter naps and is getting too demanding during the day for me to concentrate on a letter. The only reason I can write you now is that Rich has taken M to L.A. to see his dad.

The sky is filled with smoke today and there is an orange-colored haze to the light, all from those terrible fires a couple of hundred miles from here. I am stunned that the smoke is so great that we can actually see it here. Poor Sierras (and am I glad we took our vacation before all the fires started)!

Love,
Barbara

SEPTEMBER 11, 1987

Dear Barbara,

It has taken me a long time to write this letter because I didn't want to tell you the latest, and yet I knew I couldn't write without doing so. We have had another crash.

I think I told you that soon after we returned from Albuquerque we began getting new leads. We were exhausted and vulnerable, but still unwilling to let anything get by. One of the many seemed promising. We never met the birthmother, but Ken was in constant contact with her father. We told no one about it, and I did not tell you because I was certain you would advise that it was too soon. Well, maybe it was, maybe it wasn't—but in retrospect, I would probably do it again. The baby was born (in New Jersey, the lead through my aunt) on August 21; on August 22 birthmother signed preliminary papers; and on the morning of the 23rd we flew east and went directly to the hospital.

We arrived at 11:00 A.M. and were instructed to wait in the lobby. At 11:20, when nothing had happened, Ken called the nurses' station, and we were again told to wait. This continued until 12:30, when the birthmother's lawyer finally arrived on the scene to say no deal, she's changed her mind. We cried our way back to Milwaukee by 4:00 P.M., with diaper bag and car seat in tow. The following morning I started my new job.

Since then, I've decided that experience does not make you less vulnerable, but working certainly helps you recover more quickly. I am glad to have this job. Our leads have dried up at the same rate our bills have piled up, and my paycheck is a necessity if we are to try again. And yes—we will try again—and again and again. Don't worry about me, I am intact, though perhaps in denial (but can you be in denial if you think you might be?).

Lutheran Social Services called and asked me to write a brief article on independent adoptions, so I guess three times makes you an expert. Funny, wasn't it only awhile ago you were telling me how it's done? So, what comes around, goes around—once again.

Your birthday card was special. Thank you. I noted the loss of another year, but interestingly, didn't mourn; as Ken says, "I'm tired of being sad."

Write soon, sending *as usual*, all your hope and confidence.

Much love,
Lynne

SEPTEMBER 19, 1987

Dear Lynne,

Oh dammit, dammit, dammit. I am so enraged by what has happened to you . . . and by my part in it. Even by adoption standards you have had more than your "fair" (ha) share. For you I feel tired, weary of all that heartache. You must feel exhausted and despairing . . . and financially strapped too. Now will you consider a break?

This time, as you can tell, I am not a puddle of tears in your behalf. I am furious at fate; I am tired of having my friend go through so much. I am going to go out and buy your future baby another present to make myself feel better . . . and renew my faith that it is just a matter of time (dumb line: of course, it's a matter of time, but *how much?*).

I am glad for the busy-ness and money-producing aspects of your job. Use it as a drug, an escape. Lose yourself in it if you can.

Do I get a copy of the article you are writing for Lutheran Social Services?

Even though Miriam is taking longer naps, I seem to have even less free time now . . . because now that she walks, she is spreading her toys all over the house and because her increased mobility has shown her all kinds of new things to get into. Last week, I found her diaper pail upturned and poopy diapers all over the floor! And she loves to throw toys and things into the kitchen garbage pail. She is on the verge of crawling onto tables, so I don't dare leave her alone for a second. And, ego is beginning: she wants everything she sees, and if she can't have it, she jumps up and down in her new shoes and I have to keep biting my lip to keep from laughing. Nevertheless, I must be with her every second, and it is tiring.

Lots of feelings still churning around inside me, but M is waking up. Rest assured that I am in your corner no matter what, no matter how long or hard the rest of this journey is. I just want to do something to make you feel better or—better yet—to bring that baby to you.

Love,
Barbara

P.S. I had a dream about you just about the time you were in New Jersey. I dreamed you came to see me but had to make many stops along the way—Detroit, Denver, Phoenix—and had to leave clothes and things in each place. You did make it to my doorstep, no "things" left, but you and I were so glad to finally be together. I am not an interpreter of dreams, but why not see it as an omen anyway: your journey for that baby will end happily eventually . . . you just have to make some stops. You have already made three, and I will be here waiting till you make whatever other stops have to be made.

SEPTEMBER 28, 1987

Dear Barbara,

After fifteen consecutive days of rain, it is finally sunny, brisk, and wonderful. Better yet, I feel good, so it is time for a letter.

My new job is going very well. It is a smaller organization than I'm accustomed to, so I am able to make more of a significant impact.

Now that you know my professional skills are sharp, allow me to give myself one other well-deserved compliment. I look great. No doubt the difference is attributable to my lifestyle change—i.e., sweatpants and a ponytail vs. makeup, silk blouses, and Hermes scarves—but the ten pounds lost while grieving the summer away didn't hurt . . .

I sent my adoption piece to Lutheran Social Services (will send a copy later; I'm at work now), and they mentioned they were starting a "Resolve-like" support group in our area. Ken and I attended the first meeting, which was last Wednesday night. About thirty couples showed up, and, initially, it was very tense. I just can't shake the feeling that I'm in competition with all of them. It began with everyone introducing themselves and talking a bit about their lives. After twenty-eight "We're Tom and Sue and we like to camp, ski, etc.," it was no less tense when our turn came, Ken stood up, and (in Alcoholics Anonymous style) said, "Hi, I'm Ken and I'm infertile." It brought down the house, and the rest of the evening was sheer joy. What a transformation this man has made! A year ago he was convinced that infertility was "our little secret." What a change, what a year . . .

After hearing all of their stories, I am convinced that you are the exception to the rule (success on the second attempt), not us.

There have been, by the way, no new leads. We did register with a new agency in town that has no age restrictions and works on a lottery system rather than from a list, so maybe . . .

I know you're busy; write when you can.

Love,
Lynne

P.S. Happy Birthday to Miriam! How about a recent picture?

OCTOBER 4, 1987

Dear Lynne,

I am so impressed. Jealous even. I know from my own experience that trials and grief deepen character, but your last letter suggests that you have pulled it all together and have risen well above circumstance. You sound like the best you. You have reinforced my notion that you are an extraordinary person, worth knowing under any circumstances.

Your letter made me appreciate how different my life up to now would have been if somewhere along the line I had been given more self-esteem and a push in the right direction professionally. I was a very intuitive and competent teacher, but I never felt I was accomplishing anything. I would have had . . . could *have* a different life now, had I known or believed that I could make changes in the world. How blessed you are to believe in yourself professionally, to have work that is more than just "busy-ness" until the baby comes.

The dress arrived early, so we didn't allow ourselves to open it until the big day. Thank you so much for remembering. The blue is perfect for M's eyes, which border on navy themselves. And if shopping for the dress gave you pleasure, I am doubly pleased.

I've enclosed a letter from Planned Parenthood. Their offices generally do not refer prospective adoptive parents, but this one does. I came in contact with Kate Lim last year about a lead that my fellow had-a-baby-taken-back adoptive mother Shelley Jefferson passed on to me. We weren't chosen, but I have since heard of other leads (and babies) through Kate. I did talk with her on the phone, and she seems to understand the adoption world and sounded like she might function as a pretty good counselor. So send her a personal cover letter along with whatever picture and letter you are sending out. Then give her a call in a month or so, to let her know you are still interested and available. In your cover letter be sure to tell your long story; it'll help. Send back Kate's letter to me, as we want to contact her when it is time for baby number two.

M's birthday is—or was—terrific. My friend Kathy could not come to the party we gave, so she gave a little one for us. Then we had one here last weekend with lots of babies and toddlers and balloons and cake and ice cream and presents. Rich's dad drove up from L.A. to be here, his first trip since his wife died. It was a nice weekend. Next weekend the baby group is having a party: eight babies and sixteen proud parents all in one place. Should be wild!

On her birthday itself, we toasted Miriam in champagne and, after she went to bed, we reread the Miriam Chronicles—a diary Rich wrote from the time we started the adoption process until we got Miriam. I remembered calling your home from the airport when Miriam was born and having a conversation with Ken. As I read through the story of our ordeal, I had to wonder how one body could have tolerated so much emotion and exhaustion. But I did . . . and you will too.

As to your last letter, I insisted on reading to Rich the description of the LSS "AA" meeting where Ken broke the ice. I've decided you got the husband you deserve: he has grown, as has his love, as much if not more than you. I am a fan. What a helluva great time he is going to have raising a child *this* time: he will appreciate and relish every second, I'll bet.

I am intrigued by the LSS meeting. Why SO many people? Do you like the leader? Why didn't she or he ask for more infertility-centered information? (I'll never forget the first meeting of our pre-adoption group when we listened to one heartrending story after another.) How will the next sessions be run? Well, now you have a great network of people who will support you and whom you can support in the trials ahead. Let me tell you, supporting others is one of the most healing things you can do for yourself. (You didn't think I wrote these long letters because I *like* you, did you?)

The five-by-seven is a copy of our official adoption-day photo. I have been waiting since April to send it to you when I thought you would be in a "good place." It is a symbol of my greatest victory over adversity, self-defeat, and depression. I hope it offers you hope and courage, as should the miniature Japanese statue I'm sending. It is supposed to symbolize both hope and courage.

Love,
B.

OCTOBER 24, 1987

Dear Lynne,

I've already written you about my fantasy invention, the remote-control typewriter which can be attached to your brain and types whatever you are thinking. Once it becomes a reality, you will be receiving letters from me just about every day. I talk to you when I am watching Miriam, when I am in the shower, when I am walking down the street with her on my back, and so on. The trouble is, she becomes more demanding . . . and requires watching more closely each day, and nap times are getting shorter and, AGH, I am frustrated at not writing to you more often. I know you understand, but I don't like it: I know from my own response to an empty mailbox that silence can be misinterpreted. Rest assured I write to you a great deal more than you ever receive.

In fact, the reason I am able to sit down and write a long, juicy letter today is that Rich is taking Miriam for the whole weekend. Right now they are on a long stroll somewhere. They spent the morning at a local toddlers' gym. And tomorrow I am going out: to hike alone and to see if Macy's has any slacks in my size.

The reason he has number-one responsibility for her all weekend is because last week I was a single parent for five days while he was in Portland. (By the way, *when* you get your child, you will immediately resolve—though I know you have already—that this marriage is forever: being a single parent is *hard!*)

You say you can't shake the feeling that you are in competition with the other couples at LSS. Well, yes you are, of course. I ended up letting go of those feelings when a woman in my adoption group shared a lead with me. We were both in competition for the same baby, and neither of us got it because we are both Jewish. And I realized that if a birthmother is involved in the process—and that is the only kind of adoption I wanted or want—she will not choose the first couple that comes along, she will choose the one that fits her criteria . . . whether that means only people who live in the suburbs or drive an American car or have dark hair or love cats or . . . God knows. We ended up competing for leads with two other couples we knew (Mary Ellen—remember her?—got the lead and the baby) and somehow it didn't bother me . . . funny, considering how competitive I can be. Oh well, don't worry about it. In the long run, it doesn't matter much. There is an infinity of possible combinations of leads and adoptive parents . . . it all works out: if you can stand the heat and the damn wait. . . .

OK, chutzpah department: I confess that I asked Ellen to send you her materials (she will not talk to anyone unless they have read her brochure already). After you get it and have read it, will you *PLEASE* consider giving her a call and joining her service? She has leads all over, she had done adoptions in Wisconsin, she is informative to talk to, and she knows the business. It could all be done by phone and wouldn't entail too much time or effort above what you are expending these days. And . . .

Well, I'll shut up. It's not worth the loss of our friendship to me to try to force you to do something you do not want. I won't say another word on the subject. But, do think about it.

Miriam is beginning to *understand,* and it is astounding to actually have a "conversation" with her. "Miriam, get the ball and give it to Mommy . . . Throw the ball . . . Where is your doggie? . . . That's right . . . Bring Mommy the doggie." It is a trip to watch her listen intently and try to understand what we are saying. We are even having to start to spell out certain words we don't want her to understand. We are berserkly excited about this development.

Latest statistics: twenty-two pounds (seven and a half at birth a year ago) and thirty and three-fourths inches tall (twenty-one at birth). The most amazing year of our lives . . . not to mention hers.

Someday you and I will write letters exchanging facts and advice and discussion only about our little darlings. In the meantime, rest assured that I NEVER hold Miriam on my shoulder when she is asleep (just before I put her in her crib) without thinking of you with love and saying to you, "Hold on, friend, hold on. It's worth it. All of it, it's worth it."

My love,
Barbara

NOVEMBER 6, 1987

Dear Barbara,

Two interesting things have happened since I last wrote. First, LSS has taken pity on us and agreed to place us on their domestic infant waiting list. This despite the fact that they had previously told us that there was no such list, since they were completely out of the domestic baby "business." Of course, I did not remind them of this, and just about kissed their feet in appreciation. We are couple number sixty-three within the state of Wisconsin. Last year forty-nine babies were placed, SO maybe by 1989. Sounds far away, but at least it is something.

The second interesting occurrence is the arrival on the scene of birthmother number four (named Kathryn). She called us after being referred by the Albuquerque attorney who worked with Carrie. She is twenty-three years old, bright, bold, and I think, brash. I won't bother now with all the details of "her story" because the interesting part is ME. I have changed, I am back in control, and I will not allow myself to be manipulated simply because there might be a baby involved. Kathryn wondered why she should choose us; I asked why we should choose her. She told me she "might" be interested in annual contact after placement; I told her that was out of the question. She said she would like to choose the baby's name; I told her that I would choose MY baby's name. I guess what I am trying to tell you is, I have learned (FINALLY) what you, my friend, have been trying to tell me. Kathryn continues to call us and we talk, but we are not vested in anything with her to date and won't be, if we cannot come to some major agreements. Of course, I will keep you closely informed.

Work continues to go well.

At home, we continue to renovate ourselves into a frenzy. I must send you some new pictures; the house has really come along.

I'm looking forward to Thanksgiving—we are spending it alone. A welcome relief.

Well, must wrap this up.

Love,
Lynne

NOVEMBER 12, 1987

Dear Lynne,

Do you remember the Texas scam artists (the married couple who wanted us to move them to California and set them up in an apartment)? I wrote then how great it felt to say no. I told you how that experience taught me the importance of taking as much control as you can in an adoption.

But that was then and this is now. I am a lot less angry and more able to see adoption from more than one side. I still feel strongly that we adoptive couples should not allow ourselves to be steamrolled by the demands of birthmothers, out of fear that if we don't do everything they want, we will lose the baby. That is no way to establish what may very well be a lifelong relationship. However, neither should we feel that only our concerns and needs count.

Your last letter reminded me of the way I felt when we were dealing with that couple. You have been hurt—over and over and over. Once again you find your fate in someone else's hands, and you resent it. So, you strike back. But please, Lynne, for just a moment try to step back and see the whole picture.

The hard truth is that in adoption the baby is never entirely yours. Would that it were so. You are never just like other families. I think you need to come to terms with that reality.

I feel a good adoption requires a measure of trust, of negotiation on both sides. You have to give just as much as you have to draw the line clearly so the birthmother knows your limits. And you have to take yet another risk, dammit. You cannot take complete control, as much as you would like to.

I was dragged unwillingly into a relationship with Lily. I didn't think I could tolerate not knowing what was going to happen . . . again. My friends and family were concerned only for me and, so, encouraged my attitude of "just give me the baby and go away."

It was Lily who taught me that this adoption is not just about us and our passionate desire for a baby. One day I couldn't bear the anxiety a moment longer, so I wrote her a letter. I told her it was from my heart to hers, that no one else knew I was writing it. I said that she had the power to quite destroy me if she were to change her mind after I saw the baby. I didn't think I could survive the blow. I asked her—begged, really—to think hard about what she was doing. I told her that she could change her mind at any time until we got on the plane and it would be okay, but please not after that.

She wrote back that she recognized what a great risk I was taking by going through open adoption all over again. But did I recognize the risk *she* was taking? Did I know that *everyone* in her town, everyone in her church, everyone in her family was telling her that she was making the biggest mistake of her life? That "those folks from San Francisco" would take the baby and never be heard from again? That all the promises she had heard meant nothing, would mean nothing, in a court of law once the adoption was final?

Well, I was humbled. Till then I really hadn't thought about the trust she had placed in us. After that it was a lot easier to like, and then love, Lily.

I'm afraid what I've written will make you angry. Please understand I write to you in response to your pain, and in remembrance of my own. I think of you every day, and every day I hope that when the letter carrier comes there will be a letter from you.

With love,
Barbara

Barbara,

I've just finished reading your letter and you were right—I'm angry! I am beginning to think you have become as narrow-minded about "open" adoption as the traditionalists are about "closed." Open adoption, of course, sounds good, but let's face it, the jury will be out until this generation of babies are grown. Perhaps, despite everyone's best intentions, the various relationships involved will result in significant problems that today cannot even be anticipated.

I think meeting a birthmother and having a relationship with her is critical—but the nature of that relationship is personal and different for everyone. I think being honest with your child about his or her birthmother (and anything else you know) is essential, and I would certainly assist in any meeting he or she might someday pursue—but in my own heart of hearts I do not believe postplacement contact is in *anyone's* best interest. I think it is absurd to say that a birthmother chooses open adoption so that her baby is not "gone forever." With or without contact, the baby *is* in fact gone—and that is sad—so sad—but it is the way it is.

When Carrie's baby was born, she screamed and said, "I love her, but I can't keep her," and I stood there and wept. Everyone assumed they were tears of joy, but they were not—I truly ached for Carrie. So I do understand (as much as I'm able) the birthmother's feelings. To make it as easy as possible, I will jump through some hoops—but not every hoop, not anymore. Some things are not negotiable, they are personal—not right, not wrong—and if my issues cost me a baby, so be it. I have worked through my pain and grief, but working through it doesn't mean it all goes away. I don't know if you still have your pain, but let me remind you that it regularly screamed out from every letter—until Miriam. In the end, I think that is truly the only cure.

My anger will go away; I know you wrote as my friend. No doubt the hurt will also subside—but for tonight, just tonight, you have become one of those women who *has* a baby, and I am still one who does not.

Lynne

NOVEMBER 28, 1987

Dear Lynne,

Well, I am chastened. Your angry letter was very clear on where you stand and what you will and won't accept in open (in quotes) adoption. Some I knew, some I didn't, and some was just plain miscommunication between us.

When you wrote, "Future contact is out of the question," I think you assumed I understood that to mean *in person* contact. I didn't; I assumed you meant contact of any kind, ever—in other words, closed adoption. I figured any birthmother whom you encountered outside of an agency would be unwilling to do that. Now I understand. And, as you will see below, I definitely agree with your feelings that way-down the line contact is OK (maybe you wouldn't even object to letter writing; I don't know), but not "drop in anytime—just think of it as OUR child." Agreed!

I think we are at different levels of openness, and you are right to point that out. I think I do or will try harder to respect our differences. Nevertheless, I do want you to know that I feel strongly that open adoption is healthier all around, for the parties concerned when it happens and for the adopted child as she or he grows. I am strongly of the opinion that the less kept in the closet the better, in *any* interpersonal situation.

I really appreciated your comment that I am as narrow-minded about open adoption as the "other side" is about closed. It stung because it is accurate, and accurate about me in general. When I am converted (a very rare occurrence; I am too cynical), I can become the worst of the true believers. A fault, and one reinforced by Rich, who is even more that way . . . and even more cynical and therefore harder still to convert. We have been to too many workshops, lectures; read too many books; talked to too many adoptees—adult ones—and adoptive parents and birthmothers. We believe strongly, and therefore can become insensitive to others' beliefs. For that I apologize. Nevertheless, I still believe what I believe . . .

. . . Which doesn't mean dealing with the reality of open adoption is easy for me. We got a card yesterday from Lily, the first in months. She has asked for seven days off from work around Xmas, and "we plan on coming out to see all of you." Rich and I spent most of yesterday in a fog, feeling distant from Miriam and very anxious and worried about the visit. I knew Lily would come out once (to corroborate that she had made the right decision, as many birthmothers seem to need to do), and I guess it is better sooner than later, but it feels later right now! Her being here will bring—has already brought back—feelings that we had begun to forget: we *are* infertile, we are NOT M's biological parents, Lily is an important person in her life. Miriam won't remember it; and we will recover . . . but still I think of it as very stressful. We are scared.

Of course, we had already made our holiday plans to go to L.A. to see the grandparents right after Xmas. We have no idea just when she is coming, whom she'll be with, where we will put them up, how much time they will spend here, and HOW WE WILL COPE! It is great comfort to know that this bothers Rich as much as me. I am hoping the only time she can come is when we will be in L.A. and, therefore, the whole thing will fall through. Ain't I gutsy? Will keep you posted. In the meantime, I am asking my friends to start collecting Valium for me.

Let me know how your lead with birthmother number four is going, how your Thanksgiving vacation was, what your Xmas plans are, and *do you have any Valium?*

Love,
Barbara

Dear Lynne,

Your picture stares out at me daily, and daily I wonder what is going on. Half of me is convinced you've become so angry at me that you've decided to forget the whole friendship. Half of me feels silence isn't your style, that maybe the Xmas rush (yours, the post office's) has delayed your letter.

I am mystified (did I again anger you in my last note?), sad, and hurt. What's going on? Are we friends? Please let me know.

I hope you are OK and that you have a good holiday time.

In friendship,
Barbara

DECEMBER 22, 1987

Barbara,

Waited in line for twenty tension-filled minutes with hordes of Christmas maniacs so I could mail your already very late gift. I waited and I pushed and I shoved and I inquired sweetly as to whether there was a shorter line for Hanukkah parcel post, *but I waited* because I didn't want you to think that I'd forgotten or, worse, was still mad. Then I got home and there was your card hoping I wasn't "still mad." "Oy," said the shiksa with the Yiddish bent, "mad is what I wasn't, before I got to the damn post office."

It is a difficult time of year—another holiday without, another empty milestone. Birthmom number four gone—no regrets—better now than later. We have placed all bets on LSS. In addition to the traditional program we are in with them, we have been told there is another avenue to pursue. It seems they keep a file of letters or resumes for birthmothers written by prospective parents who want "open" adoptions. To date, they (LSS) have not had a lot of interest, but we immediately sent them our stuff. Interesting—but still we wait. Why is it in regard to waiting that experience makes it harder, not easier. Sorry for myself? You betcha!

My parents up from Florida on the 25th—Ann here on the 26th—lots of bodies—hopefully all distracting.
Falalalala

Love,
L.

JANUARY 4, 1988

Dear Barbara,

Two gifts from you on the same day. Thank you so much. The basket from Central America was special, as was the long-awaited Japanese statue. The latter now sits on my desk, right beside my favorite picture of you and Miriam (the homecoming). As always, you are so thoughtful. I'm afraid my Hanukkah gift to you was not nearly so creative. Forgive me; it was hard to conjure up much enthusiasm for the season. I am not depressed, though very glad that all the parties and assorted celebrations are over.

I need to write you a long letter and tell you everything that is happening, but until then the bottom line is LSS. Have I told you all this? We're on their waiting list and their "EZ" payment plan, and they *guarantee* placement. Ken has convinced me that this "bird in the hand" is the way to go, and I agree it is smart and practical, but it is so hard to ignore the leads that keep coming our way. Many have sounded good, but none has come without a $5,000 price tag, and we simply can't do both. So we wait—Ken, ever so calmly; me, tearing my hair out. . . . I am convinced LSS will go belly-up the day before we are to get our baby.

A long, quiet weekend awaits with lots of time for a long letter to you. 'Til then—

Love,
Lynne

JANUARY 9, 1988

Dear Lynne,

Happy New Year . . . all of it. May it be a happy one for you during the waiting (it's possible if you indulge yourself and keep your belief in the happy ending), and may the happiness continue into the dream come true.

Needless to add, I am more than a little relieved to hear that we are still friends. An empty mailbox is easy to interpret, and boy was I interpreting! I am also feeling optimistic about your future. After our heated exchange I came away with a clearer understanding of where you stand and what you can stand . . . and LSS sounds like the right solution for you. This way, no matter how endless and infuriatingly SLOW the wait, at least *you know it will end happily.* That is the only advantage of waiting for an adoption, over waiting for a pregnancy or a test or a period or whatever.

I too am relieved that the holidays are over, but then I always am . . . baby or no baby. Jews often feel culturally isolated and culturally threatened in December, and having a baby in a "mixed" marriage doesn't make it easier. Last year I decided I could no longer deal with the stress of present exchange; besides the self-imposed pressure of getting just the right gift, I also felt almost coerced into participating in Xmas, which I resent . . . in spite of a supportive and basically pagan husband (who insists on a Hanukkah bush as a pagan symbol). So this year you were the only adult, besides Rich, to whom I gave a present. Giving to kids and babies (mostly Hanukkah presents) is easier and such fun that I don't mind at all. God willing (Zeus? the Druids? St. Elizabeth? all of them?), next Xmas we will send presents only to each other's child! And if I haven't said it before, thank you for last Hanukkah: your shower of gifts was truly wonderful right in the midst of all the Baby's First Xmas stuff. (I know that must be painful to read. Excuse me.)

The calendar is lovely. Somehow I guess you knew that we are birders, Rich a serious one. It also goes perfectly with the book on the Western flyway I gave Rich. Listen: I was so thrilled to get a gift from you, thereby ending the silence I was getting anxious about, and it came on Xmas eve. WHEW!

I am pleased that your gifts arrived and tickled that they came on the same day. I am especially touched at what you have done with the Japanese netsuke. You have such elegant taste; I can just visualize how it looks on a desk. Nevertheless, that is the last time I order anything from that catalog. Three months late is a bit much.

Well, Lily did not come for Xmas, only sent us a card which said "Hope to see you real soon." We have decided there is no point in obsessing about it. But we both feel there is a visit in our future. I just don't know. My initial hysteria has simmered down, largely because everything is so uncertain. I have no way of guessing how it will feel at the time, but I have no doubt BOTH of us will feel temporarily distant from Miriam, and that feeling and all the anxiety and stress will rapidly dissipate after Lily *et al.* are gone. It is hard to be philosophical when I know it will be hard, hard, hard on me.

Miriam is astounding, perched right at the beginning of the terrible twos (they are supposed to start around eighteen months). We are heavy into NO NO NO these days, and I am dealing with the struggle I knew I would have—not wanting to be too repressive with her but needing to set limits. She is now just over thirty-two inches (I marked it on the growth chart you sent me), which is almost half my height. Amazing!! She talks too: what an explosion. Almost overnight it seems. I have been compulsively writing down new words, acquired in just over a month. My favorite, of course, is "Mama." There are other kinds of amazing breakthroughs, almost daily. Today she figured out how to buckle her belt on the highchair (if she figures out how to unbuckle it, we are in TROUBLE). She has just mastered pulling her pull toys and sitting on her horse-with-wheels and making it go down the hall. She also loves to do precisely what we have told her NOT to do (open the fridge, touch the stove) over and over and over, all the while saying "no, no, no." I am struggling: either to bite my lip to keep from laughing or to control my temper.

I'm enclosing a few photographs of our visit to my parents. You get to see our blue-eyed beauty in her holiday finery and some of Dad's paintings in his studio.

It is a quiet Sunday afternoon, and somehow I bet you, too, are sipping a cup of tea and writing me. Nice thought. If you are sitting in that stunning cream-colored chair with the little mahogany table, decanter, and two glasses nearby (GREAT fabric on the chair), just remember to *enjoy* it while you can. Soon enough the table, the decanter, the glasses, and the plant will have to go . . . childproofing.

I look forward to hearing from you soon. If our letters cross, you might want to be the one to write next . . . sitting at the typewriter is only possible now when M is asleep. She is very interested in "typing," and her naps are getting *shorter!*

Love,
Barbara

JANUARY 15, 1988

Barbara,

The pictures of Miriam are wonderful—thank you! She is truly a gorgeous child—and those eyes—I can't believe they've stayed so blue. Please, never hesitate to send photos or write developmental updates— I love it because she is yours and because it reinforces the notion that someday there will be a mine! Infants are precious and sweet, but the age I like the best of all is the almost-two's. They're so curious and brave at that age. I also like that funny little toddling kind of walk— what a great 1988 you are going to have.

Your comments regarding LSS are right on—they are slow, steady, and safe. Ken thinks it is the ideal solution, "no emotional upheavals; all we have to do is wait." I think it is mostly slow. Being on their list does not mean we will rule out all independent leads; however, we will have to be very selective.

I'm so glad that it is January and time to get on with real life; the holidays did me in this year. Like you, I'm burned out on mandatory gift giving. Christmas at our house is usually a capitalistic nightmare, but not this year. I gave Ken a book and a sweater, and he gave me high-topped white Reeboks—just what I wanted! My parents were here from Florida and left just before we all drove one another crazy. I know they both feel my pain, but their reactions to it are very different. My father simply does not know what to say, while my mother, on the other hand, cannot stop talking. She follows

me everywhere, telling me inane stories about relatives I barely remember and their children, operations, and problems. I think I've
mentioned before that she also has a huge collection of infertile and
adoption stories that she can call up at a moment's notice. "Remember
Helen, Aunt Jane's sister's daughter? Well, she tried to get pregnant
for years. The doctor said it would never happen but *blah blah blah*—"
this all shouted outside the bathroom door where I've escaped for
privacy and a bath. So anyway, I was relieved when the visit was over.
I assume you spent time with your family in December, based on the
photos you sent with your last letter—how did that go? And do tell
about Xmas eve with the in-laws. Your father is a very talented artist.
Is this a hobby or profession?

Must wrap this letter up and head for a meeting. . . . I'm really
comfortable in our new town now and hopeful that we'll stay put.
More soon.

Love,
L.

JANUARY 27, 1988

Dear Lynne,

Sometime in some letter—I can't seem to find it—you mentioned that
with LSS you are guaranteed a child by such and such a date. Am I
right? If so, when? I recollect 1989, but hope I am wrong, that it is
sooner. What is that saying? "Life is what happens while you're waiting
for yours to start," or some such thing. I hate the fact that we have to
wait so long for your child, hate it not nearly so much as I imagine
you hate it. However, it is sounding more and more in each letter that
you are coping very well and making the time count. The holidays
are always the worst, remember. We've got nowhere to go but up and
into spring. That was always a comfort to me during my interminable
wait—the seasons change, and warmth, blue skies, and flowers inevitably return.

Love your gift exchange with Ken. It sounds so thoughtful and sensible, none of that how-much-money-can-I-spend syndrome. Did I tell you Rich and I bought ourselves our first piece of folk art—a sensational Mexican mask—wooden. The head of a man carved to look like a fish, waves in the beard, and a "tail" of sorts in the hair and scales on the cheek and small fish for eyebrows. Sounds weird, I know, but it's compelling. We call him *pescadore* (fisherman). The minute we walked into the dealer's showroom, we knew he was what we wanted. Anyhow, there really is no place to put him here, so we will simply have to move to find a place to put him in!

Christmas at Rich's dad's, as you requested: We flew down Christmas morning with Miriam. Now, even a one-hour flight with a fifteen-month-old can be harrowing—having her stay *anywhere* without running about is a challenge. So by the time we had dealt with the plane trip and luggage and the car ride to Dick's house, Miriam was pretty tired and bewildered and overstimulated. We walked into the living room where the whole family was gathered.

I put Miriam down and, as I did, noticed that, in spite of my request, the house had not been childproofed. She headed for the tree (oy) and the crystal knicknacks and then all the candy and dips on the low coffee table (double oy). And so it went, with Rich and me taking turns corralling and/or diverting her.

Anyhow, she finally went over the edge into a tantrum. I took her into the bedroom to calm her down and try to get her to take a bottle, thereby missing the big dinner.

I appreciate your encouragement and reassurance about writing about Miriam. I still feel uneasy about that. This is your favorite age, you say. Yes, the toddler walk is delightful, and the explosion of language is stunning. I have loved every age, and the current one is always the best. But a bit of reality here: This is also the age of the terrible twos. I thought they started at twenty-four months, but everyone says they are usually over by then. Miriam is just starting—mostly throwing herself on the ground and screaming when we tell her she can't have something. The "NO NO NO" and "mine" stages are just around the corner. So I am treasuring each delicious day. And they ARE delicious. She has begun imitating: her Doggie has to be fed and diapered and put to sleep and kissed and hugged. It is beautiful beyond words to see her act out the care and love we have shown her. She loves to wipe the floor with a rag (poor babe, her mom is a compulsive cleaner) and wants to shave like dad and wear my shoes. The capper to everything, though, is when she comes up to me and jabs me with her index finger and says "mama" and then hugs my knees. OY, the tears. I have cried more in joy in the last month than I did the *first* month.

She is also incessantly demanding—I cannot go to the bathroom alone without having her try to drag me off the toilet to play. It is draining and hard . . . and hard to keep my patience and hard to discipline in a calm, loving way. I want to do a good job, and I finally see that this is the time to get some child care on a regular basis. I am hoping to do some trading and also hire someone so that I can have at least one and a half days to myself and get a break from her. It will make me a better parent.

There she is. The nap is over. Much more to share about M in the future.

Send pictures of what you've done to your house, yes?

Much love,
B.

P.S. Yes, my dad is a professional artist—gave up premed (in 1917!) to do what he loved and has done it ever since . . . always a struggle financially, but a source of great and *rare* contentment. I'm so pleased you like his work.

FEBRUARY 7, 1988

Barbara,

It's a gorgeous Sunday—lots of sun, cold, clear, and snow-covered. So nice, in fact, that Ken and I dumped all household chores and took the afternoon off. We cross-country skied for three hours, first along the lakefront. A lot of exercise, but oh it hurts so good. . . . The serenity of the day also helped us sort through some recent happenings. There is another birthmother—actually, two: one in Albuquerque (referred by our former attorney) and one in (of all places) Wisconsin (from the LSS file I told you about)! The leads occurred within days of one another. Anyway, we're going to try to play both out. I don't want to go into all the details of each . . . birthmoms are named Terry (New Mexico) and Tracey (Wisconsin) . . . but should it go further, I will certainly tell you more. Due dates: April 24, Terry, and June 4, Tracey. I've become far too cynical to get excited, but, as ever, I am hopeful.

I have no other news and really should attack about a jillion dirty dishes in my kitchen. Last night we had friends over, and I made a dinner you could die for—veal medallions stuffed with spinach in a mustard sauce—damn, it was good!.

Next letter I'll send photos of our home improvements.

Love,
Lynne

FEBRUARY 18, 1988

Dear Lynne,

I am impressed by your Sunday, spontaneously skiing away the afternoon. It says a lot about both your marriage and your state of mind. Both sound in excellent shape. Rich was downright green with jealousy over the skiing . . . ready to move back East again. I am jealous over the time you have (that sounds insensitive; hold on) to do what you really want and damn the consequences. Cannot do that any more . . . well, not easily . . . with a child. So enjoy your freedom; sounds like your free days are numbered—and the numbers are lower than we thought.

Two leads?! Gevalt. Rich and I are rooting for the one due the 24th of April, as that is Rich's birthday. But either one will do; we're not proud. Sooner—I prefer this choice—or later this year (yes?) your dream will come true. I am beginning to dare to get excited for you again. I will get excited for you; don't you get excited. Keep that aloof, slightly dubious attitude; it will keep you sane.

Your dinner, too, sounds delicious. Remember that menu, as that's what you can fix for me when we finally meet. It will have to happen someday, screaming kids all around us.

Tonight I go to dinner with friends of a friend. They were referred to me because they are just about to jump into the adoption world. They have anxieties you and I have shared; they have questions and hostile feelings and rage that I have experienced; they have hope, too. I hope I can give them facts and feelings balanced with sensitivity—a sensitivity that I hope has grown since our recent disagreement. I will let you know.

My best to Ken. Don't forget photos of your home improvements.

B.

FEBRUARY 24, 1988

Barbara,

Tell Rich I'm sorry, but there won't be a baby on his birthday, at least not my baby. Believe it or not, WE made this decision, and though it was difficult, it feels right. Soon after I wrote to you, Terry in Albuquerque began to insist that we come out prior to the birth. She also decided that she no longer needed counseling (New Mexico state law requires only two sessions), and her counselor told me that she was being harassed at school. Terry attends a high school for pregnant students, and 95 percent of the school population is Hispanic. According to the counselor, adoption is almost unheard of in the Hispanic culture; instead, birthmothers rely on their own extended families to help them rear the child. All of this, combined with the fact that Terry is fifteen years old, made us decide to walk away. So, we're out, and I cannot and will not look back.

We have, however, recently met Tracey from Wisconsin. She is eighteen, street-smart and savvy. She seems to have a real grasp on the reality of having an infant (she babysits daily) and says that it's just not for her at this time in her life. We liked her a lot and were especially touched that she chose us because "You seem to love each other a lot, and you're so funny." Yes sir, we are hilarious . . .

Actually, I did think that was kind of nice, as a sense of humor is something that consistently draws me to people, too. I recall a letter you wrote pre–Nancy's birth. You were having some unexplained bleeding, and you included a mental news headline—something like, "Infertile woman waits years for baby, gets baby and dies." I think that is when I first knew we were, indeed, kindred spirits!

Tracey lives about forty-five minutes away from us, and we hope to see her about once a month until delivery, but I WILL REMAIN COOL, I promise! No more agonizing over every word and deed. If she does, she does, and if she doesn't, she doesn't. One lousy thing about Wisconsin—following the birth of the baby, the birthmother must wait four weeks (sometimes longer depending on the court schedule) before signing the Termination of Parental Rights agreement, and during this time the baby must be placed in a foster home AND the foster home may not be the home of the prospective parents. So IF all goes well, it won't be until July that we get the baby. Maybe your birthday?! Feels so far away . . .

I have taken, but not developed, house pictures for you. Next letter. The work, as I wrote before, has been massive. Since June we have painted every room, reglazed terra-cotta tile floor in the sun room, replaced every light fixture, replastered the kitchen walls and wallpapered, refinished upstairs and downstairs oak floors (3,000 square feet), turned an outside porch into an inside family room, and remodeled a half bath. WHEW! No wonder we're exhausted AND broke. In April we turn to the outside—more paint and lots of land-scaping. I must say, though, despite it all, I love the house and the neighborhood. We're five minutes from the lake and fifteen minutes from "downtown." We really feel settled here. Our once-frequent trips to Chicago have been reduced to quarterly visits, or whenever I need a haircut. Only one woman in the entire world knows what to do with my miserable hair.

Love,
Lynne

MARCH 9, 1988

Hello friend,

So now you're down to one lead. Your decision to drop the other one shows you and Ken are in control—well, as much as possible, and that can only be good.

Tracey in Wisconsin sounds perceptive and like she's really paying attention to who you are. I like that—reminds me in retrospect what little attention we got from Nancy. We were a convenience, but never *real* to her. Anyhow, it's a helluva long time till June/July. I hope you don't have to see her a lot and invest a lot of emotion in her.

I am optimistic that you are clearly going to survive all this—and that there will be a happy ending. As a favorite poem of mine says, just keep "plant(ing) your own garden and decorat(ing) your own soul."

I am excited and wish June/July were soon.

My evening with the couple who are about to begin the adoption process was . . . well, enlightening. I listened a lot and gave feedback and suggestions and answered dozens of serious, heartfelt questions. Still, I left feeling uneasy.

They are both brilliant and talented. He is the owner of a local popular restaurant, and she's an extraordinarily talented sculptor and college art professor—and stunning-looking, to boot. Also, the only child of deceased parents, thus passionately attached to carrying on both her bloodline and her talent.

They asked about Lily's family, and I told them . . . after prefacing my remarks with a description of the process I went through to let go of my fantasies of adopting a baby with a background similar to mine. Little headway. They're gonna get the best baby the market has to offer . . . to match their fancy Saab and home.

Sounds crass, and it made me sad.

Miriam is up to seventy-five words. Between our weekly front-window observation of the garbage truck this morning and my buying a new kitchen garbage can this afternoon, she spent the greater part of the day practicing "gargar" while nodding her head vigorously to show she knew what she was talking about. Cute? Oy, *you bet.*

Nine-thirty and I'm doing a fast fade.

My best,
B.

P.S. I'm enclosing some recent pictures of Miriam.

On March 18, 1988, Lynne received a pot of red tulips along with a note which read:

Thank you (us?) for a three year correspondence that has never failed to be enriching and a friendship, like the tulips, which deepens and blossoms with time.

My love,
Barbara

P.S. May our fourth anniversary see us corresponding about diapers and sleepless nights. Yes.

MARCH 19, 1988

Barbara,

Lately I've decided I have learned and matured and mellowed. I suspect some of my old letters would embarrass me now—filled, as they were, with all that whining about what is and isn't fair—the fact is, life isn't fair.

Still, everything I've been through will make me a better parent (and person), so I choose to believe there was and is a purpose!

Our relationship with Tracey continues to grow, primarily through her efforts. We talk on the phone at least weekly and plan for a third face-to-face meeting next weekend. Also—she wants me to be her labor coach and attend classes with her (beginning April 13). *STOP*—everything you're thinking Ken has already said, but I'm doing it anyway. I believe Tracey's baby will be mine, but should she change her mind, I will not regret my decision. It will either be a beautiful introduction to my child or the ultimate good deed for a young woman who really needs someone. I'm not so foolish that I don't know I can't be disappointed again, but I will never be hurt like I was before. Like Ken, you must trust that I know what is best for me.

The couple mentioned in your letter were certainly fortunate to have the benefit of your perspective. I have struggled, though quietly, with my own fantasies of finding a baby with a similar background to mine. I still have a few—though really not many, and I think it is because of Ann. I am only an every-other-weekend stepparent, but after five years I can truly see a little part of her that comes from me, and somehow it compensates a bit for the fact that she isn't really mine.

Does that make sense?

Love,
L.

P.S. Your anniversary card just arrived—three years, unbelievable! As always, I'm so glad we're friends.
P.P.S. Miriam gets "gorgeous-er" with every month (sigh).

MARCH 30, 1988

Dear Lynne,

Aha, I knew it! After spending hours trying to get a recalcitrant (that's putting it nicely) Miriam to take her nap, I gave up and packed us up for the zoo . . . throwing in stationery to write you "just in case." Yup, here we are in the car one block from home, and she's snoring away. So I'll put on a Mozart tape and pretend I'm relaxing and writing at the desk (and try to remember what was in your last letter).

Thanks for the photos you sent. What a wonderful house, clearly filled with character and charm, and you've certainly worked hard to bring it out. I love the sun room and living room (so much like the one of my fantasies!). You have the same outdoor furniture and Weber grill we do, by the way. Congratulations on putting together a home filled with love and lovely objects. Can't wait to hear tales of how your future wee one tears it apart.

Gleefully.

I'm finding that almost all the women I associate with regularly through the baby network are pregnant. I hadn't realized when I went around networking with new moms that there'd be a point when I'd be dealing with . . . well, I guess you'd call it my pseudo–secondary infertility. Much easier than what you're dealing with (so well) these days. I find I'm jealous of their having those amazing, miraculous first days of getting to know a newborn.

Which made me realize with a shock that I'm already feeling jealous with anticipation of what awaits you: not just the precious, astounding, and phenomenally exhausting first days, but doing it *for the first time*. Once you get through postadoption depression, it is the highest of highs. I look forward to having a newborn again, but by definition it can never be as exquisite as the first time. I hope you allow yourself the quiet realization that eventually that time of daily miracles will be yours.

Your warm, caring personality, which comes through in your letters and is a major source of my wanting to maintain this correspondence over the past three years, is what got you the lead on that baby with the birthmother in New Mexico and now Tracey. It is obvious they felt connected to you and supported by you . . . and committed to you. Tracey sounds quite involved with you (I hope more than you are with her). That's a good sign, but is she getting counseling? Because if she gives you her baby, she will then be losing the child and—in a sense—you. She'll need a cushion then.

Look, I am—once again—scared for you. But if I've learned nothing else in the last six months, it is that you have contacted your center of strength and will survive no matter what. I trust your gut instincts as I trust my own. Suffering and loss have given us that trust, I think.

Rich just returned from five days in Portland. I wish every pregnant teenager in America could have been a fly on the wall as I struggled to deal with Miriam's nonstop demands twelve hours a day. Each night I fell asleep a half hour after she did. Such hard work! To do a good job as an unassisted single mother is very, very hard.

My birthday is coming up, and it feels like a hard one. I'll be forty-five, an ugly, not-young number. (Is forty-six too old to "have" a baby? Is sixty-two too old to deal with a teenager? These are serious issues for me these days, though no one else thinks I've cause to worry.) I'd love to have you get your baby around the time of my birthday. It'd fit, somehow.

Miriam turned one-and-a-half yesterday, and to celebrate she said her 100th word (what else around Passover?: "bunny"). I'll stop writing them down now.

I'm taking a wonderful class for parents of young adopted children (on the unique issues, the "telling," adolescence, etc.). Will pass on info, bibliographies, articles when I have time.

Wishing you a joyous Passover,

Barbara

Dear Lynne,

I've written you so many times in my head over the last few weeks that I find myself surprised not to find any answer in my mail. All the letters begin, "It isn't that I'm not thinking of you . . ."

. . . it's just an astounding lack of real *free* time in my life. "I live for naptime" could be a bumpersticker. I run around making phone calls, picking up after M (she has discovered the joys of emptying six large drawers full of clothes), paying bills, making child-care trade arrangements, eating, and all the time writing to you in my head. It's frustrating: our correspondence means so much to me.

But I feel less guilty than I would have months ago, because I feel so sure about you now. If we weren't good friends and didn't get so much from our letters, I'd say you no longer need my story, my support. I have confidence in your inner security and resolve. And I am optimistic and *excited as hell* about the future you have (some) control over.

Nevertheless, I know these waiting days are a drain, and I know my letters would help. Maybe if I told you what "channel" I'm on, we could just do a Shirley MacLaine communication?

Your bond with Tracey seems to be growing. I believe in its power. It's sounding like the "ideal" open-adoption scenario I've heard so much about. . . . Everything's going right. And if it doesn't you'll survive!

So, after over a year of tripping over your baby gift almost daily (when the baby in New Mexico died, I stored the gift away where I wouldn't have to see it all the time), now *I can't find it!* I'm just superstitious/human enough to know this is a good sign; I was super-organized and planned ahead (bought it in June of '86!!), and look what it got you: nothing. The fact that I can't find it means this is gonna work out . . . and I'll have to tear the house apart (happily) looking for it. All right!

Naptime is over . . . to be continued . . .

Nineteen-month-olds are a trip. Didn't you once write that this is your favorite age? She is verbal constantly (over 150 words!), awakens, and immediately begins naming everything in sight: "Mee Mee

(Miriam), Mommy, dog, clowny, how (house), titty (kitty), bear, pen-win (penguin)," etc. Compelling to hear! She is hitting stage two, possessives: "Mee Mee cup, Mommy chair," etc. And where a few months ago she'd have to hear a word in context ten to twenty times before using it, now she can repeat a word after hearing it only two or three times. I am fascinated.

She also prefers her way, thank you. I know who invented sit-ins: mothers of toddlers. She doesn't want to go your direction? Plunk on her tushie on the sidewalk, in the store, or in a parking lot. Another bumpersticker (for this situation): "Diplomacy is the better part of parenting." I try everything: giving in, diverting, ignoring, cajoling, bribing, and then brute force (well not really: I pick her up and tickle and/or toss her around till she forgets what she was adamant about ten seconds before). Very challenging.

And the bonding! Suddenly she is so "wedded" to me (best word) that she weeps when left with Daddy, will only let me read to her or change her. (Rich is a bit sad, but understands.) It is reasonable, but strange somehow, that dependence and independence would become so powerful simultaneously.

More soon. How many weeks till the due date?

Love,
B.

APRIL 17, 1988

Hello Friend!

Since my last letter I have spent five days in Knoxville, Tennessee, with my sister and her husband and returned home just in time for "my" first Lamaze class with Tracey. A very difficult experience—fourteen future moms and dads—and us. Tracey appears healthy and still committed to adoption. We managed to get through two hours of breathing exercises and then went out for ice cream (lots of ice cream!). She is a bright and thoughtful young woman, though the "girl next door" she ain't. . . . On the way home I allowed myself the tiny luxury of a good cry—it should be me and Ken, not me and Tracey.

Off to Florida for a long weekend, when I return, it will be almost May. The last month—forever, I hope.

Love,
Lynne

MAY 16, 1988

Barbara,

I wish you lived closer. I need a friend so badly right now that I ache. We could sit at my kitchen table and have tea, and you could reassure me that everything will be okay, and even if it isn't, that I will be.

Regardless of the ultimate outcome, there is no doubt that Tracey has bonded with me. We completed Lamaze classes on the 11th, and yesterday she begged me to come to a Tupperware party that her mother was having. Can you stand it?

The "party" was attended by relatives, friends, and neighbors, and I was clearly the main attraction. As you might imagine, I was charming and even bought about $100 worth of the damn burping bowls! On the way home I cried, mainly because of the tension, which is quickly becoming unbearable.

I fully expect the birth to be this week (so does the doctor) and with that the process begins, rather than ends. There are so many things that could go wrong—Tracey's decision, of course; health issues; the birthfather, who, to date, has not been heard from.

This morning I called LSS regarding our traditional adoption group. So far, no one has had a placement, and though they still *guarantee* it, the wait could be longer than anticipated. Big deal guarantee!

So, my friend, time for *another* leap of faith—this time with my eyes open, but still afraid to crash. I'll call.

Love,
L.

MAY 19, 1988

L.,

Omygosh! I just went through your letters file and read that Tracey's due date is June 4—whew! You must be in stage-one jitters (perpetual butterflies in your stomach, jumping when the phone rings).

Well, I'm with you—I keep flipping the pages of my datebook and noting how close the date is. You will call me—any time of day or night—won't you? I'm supposed to send you calming, centered messages, I know. But I don't feel calm.

For you, though, I do feel strong. Confident, too.

My love and company are sent your way.

Hold tight.

B.

MAY 24, 1988

Barbara,

Waiting is a lonely business. It sounds so passive, but it takes all of my time and every scrap of my energy. I am totally self-absorbed and find any unrelated conversation or work an intrusion. I research the signs of labor, review relinquishment statistics, and check in with Tracey. And I talk to Ken—oh how I talk to Ken—hours on end, until

I see the veil of concern and fear settle on his face. He doesn't say anything, but I know that he is weary of my obsession and afraid of what another crash will do to us. So it is my turn to be comforter— a new role, but one that seems to infuse me with strength. We will be okay. I will call.

Much love,
Lynne

P.S. If you can stand one more book on infertility and adoption, please read *Motherless Child* by Jacquelyn Mitchard. It is closer to my story than anything else I've seen. Second marriages, Illinois, Wisconsin, even a stepdaughter.

JUNE 10, 1988

Barbara,

My son (did I really write that?) was born at 3:00 P.M. Sunday on June 5. Tracey called us at 10:00 P.M. on Saturday night to say she was on her way to the hospital. We politely informed our two dinner guests that there would be no dessert and made it to the hospital by 11:00 P.M. It was a long and exhausting fifteen hours, but I was there for every bit of it—I even cut the umbilical cord! As you can see by the enclosed pictures, he is gorgeous! We are thrilled, excited, and scared to death.

Tracey was discharged on Tuesday, the 7th, and before she left, she had a few moments alone with the baby and her mother. I stood outside the door but couldn't help overhearing her say, "I didn't expect to love you, but I do." Then they took the baby back to the nursery, and I walked Tracey down to her mother's car. She never shed a tear, but I know she is grieving. She says talking to me and seeing my joy helps. On Wednesday the baby went to the foster family, and they have agreed to let us visit him on Sunday. Next week the birthfather will meet with the social worker. Assuming all goes well, homecoming could be by July 20.

Oh, Barbara, they just *can't* take him from me now.

Lynne

JUNE 20, 1988

Barbara,

I'm worried.

Everything was going so well until this week. Tracey has settled back into her old life, the baby is thriving with his foster family (we've visited three times), and the birthfather was scheduled to "sign off" on the 17th—but he didn't show. He has also not returned any of our social worker's many calls. It may mean nothing, of course, or it may mean everything. At best, he has stalled the entire process; at worst, he will fight for custody, and Tracey will be forced to keep the baby. I am a wreck. We will give him one more week to make contact, and if we still hear nothing, a court order will be served. Ken says I'm overreacting, and I pray that I am—but there is an icy feeling in my stomach that is all too familiar. . . .

When discussing this situation with a "friend," she said, "Well, be careful, don't get attached to the baby," and I wanted to scream, "It's too late, I'm attached, he is mine!" I know you understand that— why can't anyone else?

Okay, time to relax, do some breathing, and maybe drink a glass of wine. Letters should not be written while in the middle of an anxiety attack.

Send some positive vibes my way, and don't you dare uncross those toes yet.

Love,
L.

JUNE 24, 1988

Lynne,

First I got nervous because the envelope didn't say "Do Not Bend." Then I got nervous when your letter began "I'm worried." Oh no, I thought, surely enough is enough! Now what?

The birthfather. Ah yes, the bugaboo of just about every adoption, except ours (plural). I *don't* think you're overreacting (I'd still rather have you worried than confident until we have a real sure thing here). And I won't tell you to try to keep your emotional distance (impossible after the first warm skin-on-skin contact anyhow). But I do want to offer some reality testing here . . . if the court order you mentioned hasn't made all of this moot.

The guy—like so many other young, hormone-driven, macho birthfathers—has not been there much, right? I mean, was he concerned about prenatal care? Was he at any doctor appointments? At the hospital? Has he visited Tracey? The foster home? Has he shown any interest in the baby?

Much cooler for a young dirt bag to boast of his conquest but deny the seriousness and the responsibility. That's what his unresponsiveness to requests says to me.

I know you're worried. I worry too. You should worry, but you should also know how many adoptions I know of in which the birthfather waited until the last possible minute to sign off his rights— or was never found at all. It means acknowledging the responsibility . . . and the loss.

Let's see: Mona and Steve, Suzanne and David, Betsy and Mark still waiting it out; Karen and Dave in Oregon, Sol and Kathy, Norma and Brock never did "find" him, nor did Ruth and Glenn. You're in good company.

This doesn't mean it's "gonna be fine." If we haven't learned the meaninglessness of statistics by now, we haven't learned anything. You could be the second exception. The only one I know of is Helen and husband. The birthfather was a wealthy middle-aged married man from Beverly Hills. He fought for custody. They took him to court and won.

Good, go ahead and worry. It'll keep your feet on the ground. I'm a little nervous too, and I have to say I won't relax till the time is up and it's final. But it's Tracey I'd worry about. (I think she sounds solid and determined, but she's a female, and *those* hormones and that heartrending grieving I understand.)

My toes cramp periodically, but it's worth it.

Any "final" day set yet? It better be before my birthday. That's the only gift I want from Wisconsin this year.

Holding tight with you.

B.

JUNE 29, 1988

Barbara,

You may uncross *one* toe—he signed!!! Our wonderful social worker was tenacious, and after eighteen unanswered calls and three letters, she got him. He did everything he needed to *and* provided a complete medical history. Needless to say, we are thrilled! I know, I know, it still isn't over, but we're so damn close I can smell the Johnson's baby powder!

Tracey remains rock solid. I'm not sure if I have told you, but even during delivery she never seemed to waver. Her labor pains were sporadic until Sunday morning when they finally administered petocin to speed things up. She received no pain medication, and the entire process appeared excruciating. Her mother stood on one side of her bed, and I stood on the other. She asked me to rub her stomach, and after one really tough contraction she looked up at me and said, "I'm never going to do this again for you, Lynne." She is currently vacationing in Las Vegas—but we've kept in touch. She has many plans for when she returns, including going back to her old job and a date with an old pre-pregnancy boyfriend. She asks about the baby, of course, but we seem to spend much more time talking about ourselves. The relationship I've developed with this young woman is one I never could have imagined. There is a fourteen-year age difference, and we live in entirely different worlds, yet now—and I suspect forever—we are connected.

The court date for Tracey's "termination of parental rights" should be set by the end of the week. We've been told to expect the date to be July 19—and even I can deal with three weeks of waiting. Hell, it's less than a cycle with Clomid. After the court hearing we will all (Tracey, her mother, me, Ken, and our social worker) meet somewhere to say goodbye—Tracey's mother's idea and an excellent one. Like Tracey, her mother has been strong in her feelings that adoption is for the best—though I know she would have supported any decision Tracey had made. Funny, but I will miss Tracey. As impossible as it may sound, I love her, and I know she feels the same way about us. She wrote us a beautiful letter saying she hoped someday to be as "strong and good" as me, and I cried because the truth is, she already is the stronger one.

You've made no comments on the baby pictures I've sent, and I assume it's because you're still being cautious for me. That must be it, because he is clearly the most handsome child in the world—so tell me already!

> With hopes soaring,
> Lynne

JULY 2, 1988
(countdown: 17 days)

Lynne,

Am I excited! Oy, am I going nuts!! Just got your letter, and I'm feeling like a grandma or something (my birthday is affecting me, even at gleeful moments like this). Three years on hold—it's about time we started writing about sleepless nights, poop, and unmitigated joy. I am *ready*.

I found your package of baby stuff, another good sign. Can't wait to stand proudly in line with it at the post office. Will also send some sentimental loaners when the time is right. And will start inundating you with unasked-for advice. Oh, am I gonna have fun!

Pictures? I didn't mention? Mmm, maybe it's because I was stunned. Only Miriam looked like a "real" baby at birth, instead of a withered old bald man, like all ten other babies I know born within two weeks of her (babies of the women in my mom's group). He looks so alert and gorgeous after such a hard labor! More important, he's healthy and almost yours.

You might use your hospital connections to see if there's a new mothers' group near you that you could join. Great idea for lots of reasons: mostly it was, for me, an unbelievable high to be just another mom with a new baby. I swear I practically dripped milk that first day!

Last bit of practical advice (aren't I delightfully obnoxious?): get lots of sleep—exercise so you can sleep—and keep real busy.

I'm a little berserk here. I should continue being the cautious, conservative, experienced friend. Sorry, I've LOST IT!

Write very soon. I'm anxious to know how you are. Let me know final date for sure.

Your silly friend,
B.

JULY 8, 1988

Barbara,

The Termination of Parental Rights hearing has been set for the 26th of July—a week later than hoped for, but still so very soon. Tracey is still solid and we are ready and it is going to happen! The excitement level here is unbelievable. Mundane, domestic tasks continue but are interrupted regularly by little jumps for joy and hugs. "We're going to have a baby," we keep saying to one another, and then we take turns dancing around the house. A wonderful time filled with all the emotions I always anticipated and a couple more I hadn't. Several years ago, someone gave us a bottle of Dom Perignon that we vowed to save until baby day, and soon—very soon—I will put it on ice. On the 27th we will bring him home—and "him," by the way, will be Kenny. I wouldn't have chosen it, but it means so much to Ken, and I would never have made it to this beautiful place without my wonderful husband. The guy who said he didn't want any more children at first and could never deal with infertility treatment, let alone adoption—the guy who dances around the house now and manages to work "my son" into every conversation . . .

Right now the only minor cloud on the horizon is Annie. She, too, has gotten to the point where she believes it will happen, and sibling rivalry, with a new twist, has reared its ugly head. We have had three late-night crying sessions with her as she confesses she is scared we will love him more. She resents the fact that *his* parents will be married, that he will have only *one* home, and that he will be mine—in a way that she can't be. I think we have said all the right, reassuring things—but it does trouble me that she is so upset. Any advice?

I'm off to the store. Today's mission: car seat and crib and maybe just one teensy little adorable outfit. Eighteen days and counting.

L.

JULY 15, 1988
(twelve days and counting)

Dear Mother-to-Be,

How did two women who've never met get so close that one's state of heart is inextricably linked to that of the other? A rather wonderful surprise in our lives, due in no small part to your openness and generosity of spirit. Tracey, bless her, could no more resist you than could I. We have *all* chosen well.

Your last letter made me cry and cry with joy for you . . . and that lovely husband of yours . . . and for me, too. I'm realizing that my last bit of grief and pain is linked to yours. I've known for a long time that I wouldn't be finished till you were. And right at birthday time. I too will drink (too much) champagne to celebrate our shared births as mothers.

I have held back *so much* about parenting in spite of your wanting to hear it all. I remember and feel the pain of not having a child too intensely to just casually talk about daily events in M's development. Certainly, complaining was out of the question (you were understandably unsympathetic anyhow!).

I pray it is safe now to tell you about my private exquisite moments as a new mother . . . and how you figured in them and what I want you to do to help me purge the bits of sadness I felt and still feel. (All great moments always being bittersweet, as we've learned, no?) So . . .

Imagine a middle-of-the-night feeding (2:00 or 3:00 A.M.) when even a jammed city like San Francisco is stunningly quiet. In the almost dark, I'd slip on my robe, responding to Miriam's cry, slip into her room, and give her the bottle. Then, burp time: I'd put her on my shoulder and rock and pat till she burped. Then I'd just hold her cheek to mine and rock with my eyes closed and . . . exquisite joy. I was Mother Earth. It was and is worth everything for those moments. I'd invariably puddle up with happiness . . .

. . . and think of you. And whisper, "Lynne, hold on. Everything is worth this moment." I'd think of my sisterhood with all the other millions of mothers doing the same thing around the world, but mostly I'd think of you, realizing how much I wanted to share the joy with you and how I wouldn't rest till you were there, too.

So, promise me, at one 2:00 A.M. feeding you will hold sweet Kenny's cheek to yours and think of me. It will make me deeply content and "finished" with all the pain at last.

I look forward to babbling on and on about parenting with you for years to come.

I remember the before-the-baby-came-home ecstasy. I've never been so wild with happiness. I'm glad you're letting yourself go for it. Enjoy every second. You deserve it!

Oh, I'm getting puddly, so my writing's getting mushy too. Better stop.

Write to let me know the schedule of the 26th and 27th so I can think of you at the right time.

My love,
B.

P.P.S. Annie—I've just read all my books with sections on sibling rivalry and didn't find any discussion about a child Annie's age. I know you're saying all the right things. It is an age of grieving (seven to twelve) anyhow (more on this in years to come), so she's normal—*grieving the divorce* over again.

I'd guess it'll be mostly over before Kenny's arrival, at which time Annie can be told she's an invaluable help . . . which I bet she will be.

I know you and Ken are sensitive enough that you won't ignore her for fascination with your new baby when he arrives. I know Ken especially will remind her she is his "girl," a unique and special and first treasure. I imagine she'll need lots of that, particularly from him.

Not thoughts, just gut guesses.
M's awake—gotta go.

B.

JULY 21, 1988

Barbara,

Your last letter was beautiful. You captured perfectly the moment I have been anticipating. Mother love and the need to express it are really what this has been all about. It was in me before I was even able to define it, and upon its recognition, it consumed me. I can hardly believe that in less than one week I will hold my baby in my arms. I feel as though I know him already because I've held the hope of him for so long. I'm in love, I'm thrilled, I'm relieved. No doubt this time next week my sigh will be clearly heard even in San Francisco. It's over—finally—it's almost over.

The schedule: Tuesday, July 26, 3:45 P.M. (central standard) Tracey terminates parental rights; at 5:00 P.M. we meet Tracey and her mother for what I think will be a long dinner. Wednesday, July 27, 11:30 A.M. we pick up baby at LSS offices—home by noon—"happily ever after" to follow.

L.

JULY 27, 1988

Dear Barbara,

It's 5:00 A.M. on the morning of the 27th, and in six short hours Kenny will come home. I'm numb with exhilaration, fatigue, and if I'm honest, a little fear, too. I am a mother at last!

It seems perfectly appropriate to me that this wonderful day in my life coincides so closely with your birthday, for I truly believe today wouldn't have happened without you. Your letters sustained me for three years—you consistently gave me the courage I needed to continue, along with guidance, support, and love. Long after your baby was home, you *kept with me,* and I will forever be grateful.

I know this is a tough birthday for you, and I wish I could come up with some words to make it easier. I know only I bless the day you were born and consider you most precious. Every day I hold my sweet Kenny, I will remember you and our unique friendship that resulted in two dreams coming true.

Love,
Lynne

Epilogue

When Miriam was two and a half, we began the process again. As I had guessed, it felt quite different. The "baby lust" was considerably reduced. We worried less about our ability to survive another tragedy (we knew we could survive; we already had) than we did about the effects losing a baby might have on Miriam. Would she think she could be taken back, too?

Ellen Roseman told us that blanket mailings of letters were no longer considered effective. Now, hopeful adoptive parents were placing ads in the personal columns of newspapers. Too impersonal and too risky, we decided. So we sent out letters again, calling Ellen on a regular basis to see if she had any leads.

Five months after the letters went out, Ellen called us. "There is a young girl in Tulsa you might want to send a personal note. Her name is Destiny." I wrote her immediately. How could I keep Destiny waiting?

She was attending a continuation high school for pregnant girls. Out of the forty-five students at the school, she was one of only two or three who were even considering adoption—and the only one who followed through. Once again we found ourselves flying nervously across the country with car seat and baby bunting in tow. This time our thoughts were back home, with three-year-old Miriam—separated from us for the first time.

In the two days we spent with them in the hospital, Destiny, her supportive mother Caroline (a Forty-Niners fan like Rich), and Destiny's eight-year-old sister Patricia, became family. After the tender, bittersweet moment of tearful good-byes in the hospital room, Rich and I took our new baby girl back to our motel.

As soon as Leah fell asleep on the bed, I lunged for the phone and called Lynne.

BARBARA

Kenny was two years old when we decided we wanted to add another child to our family. We retained a local adoption attorney and had begun to reinitiate all our old leads and contacts when I met Patty. Patty was a nurse practitioner working with one of Milwaukee's fertility specialists, Dr. Charles Koh, and she spoke glowingly of his success rate.

To my surprise, I found myself dealing with many of my old issues. Parenthood was everything I'd hoped for, but I still regretted never having experienced pregnancy. My decision to return to infertility treatments was based on the fact that my treatment plan had never been completed. It had ended midterm, due to our move, and had been put on hold as we proceeded with adoption. Unlike Barbara, I had not made peace with the feeling that I had done all I could.

Our adoption search and fertility treatment were simultaneous—stressful, but not nearly as much as had been true pre-Kenny. To our amazement, I became pregnant after my first GIFT procedure (gamete intra-Fallopian transfer, a variation on In Vitro Fertilization) and on March 18, 1992, exactly seven years since my first letter to Barbara, gave birth to Daniel.

Neither of my sons came easily; they arrived only because of my overwhelming desire to mother—a desire I still don't fully understand, I only feel.

Barbara and I still have not met. Phone calls have now almost completely replaced letter writing. We share the joys and frustrations of parenthood, and we reminisce—not every time, but often—on our shared journey to this wonderful place.

LYNNE

Acknowledgments

Thanks are due to some extraordinary women who helped us learn the ropes of the publishing world: to Dorothy Wall, our first reader, for offering encouragement as well as her editing expertise; to Felicia Eth, our agent, for her energy and ability; and to Nancy Miller, our editor, for her consistent enthusiasm.

Thanks also to Patti Gebhard, who made sense out of two shoeboxes full of letters.

To all the resolute and courageous members of Resolve, thank you for teaching us about the realities of infertility and demonstrating the healing power of support.

Thanks to loyal friends: Ruth Lym, for pushing the adoption option; and to Kathy Barnhart, Sue Lowe, and Pam Vaughan for sharing what is best about women's friendship by listening and listening and listening.

To our husbands Rich and Ken, for their love and unwavering support then and now.

To Annie, who offered a first glimpse of what motherhood is all about and proved it worth pursuing.

And to Miriam, Kenny, Leah, and Daniel, without whom there would be no story.